Global Issues in Patient Recruitment and Retention

Diana L. Anderson-Foster, Ph.D.

This latest release is a collaborative effort among the following industry leaders, who generously contributed their editorial skill and subject matter expertise:

John Benbrook, MMG
Bonnie Brescia, BBK Worldwide
Felicia Fuller, DAC Patient Recruitment Services
Melynda Geurts, DAC Patient Recruitment Services
Kenneth A. Getz, Senior Research Fellow at the Center for the Study of Drug Development, Tufts University School of Medicine and founder and board chair, CISCRP
Beth Harper, Clinical Performance Partners
Joe Kim, Shire Pharmaceuticals
Marlene Llópiz, Clinica Responsable Operativa, S.C.
Rick Malcolm, Acurian
Dan McDonald, Excel Life Sciences
Sara Monday, Metroplex Clinical Research Center
Christine Pierre, RxTrials
Lacey Powers, Reata
Chris Trizna, Clinical Site Services
Kristy Wort, Acurian

CenterWatch

Global Issues in Patient Recruitment and Retention

by Diana L. Anderson-Foster, Ph.D.

Managing Editor	Cheryl Rosenfeld
Cover Design	Vaughn Anthony, Mark Gerlach
Interior Design	Holly Rose

Printed in the United States.

For more information contact CenterWatch, 10 Winthrop Square, Fifth Floor, Boston, MA 02110. Or you can visit our web site at www.centerwatch.com.

CenterWatch

10 Winthrop Square, Fifth Floor
Boston, MA 02110
www.centerwatch.com

ISBN 978-1-930624-63-4

TABLE OF CONTENTS

ACKNOWLEDGEMENTS

The undertaking of my third book for CenterWatch, as always, is both challenging and exciting at the same time. The book allows me to collaborate and connect with some of the major stakeholders, experts and renowned thinkers in the patient recruitment space. I greatly appreciate and acknowledge my co-authors' willingness to collaborate and share their knowledge. Every contributor is the best of the best!

Many thanks for the invaluable contributions and support of my colleague Felicia Fuller, who makes ideas and concepts come to life seemingly with ease! She is a brilliant writer and thinker. Thanks also go to Vaughn Anthony and Mark Gerlach for creative input and Susan Golladay for technical support.

Many thanks to Cheryl Rosenfeld for her patience in editing and attention to detail, and to Joan Chambers, who has been a part of all three recruitment publications. She is adept at coming to the rescue at the right time and place! The technical support from Imperial Clinical Research Services provided behind-the-scenes support, always a critical element in making deadlines.

Finally, special thanks to my husband John for supporting me and helping me stay on task through the many hours devoted to working on this project.

Sincerely,
Diana L. Anderson-Foster, Ph.D.

INTRODUCTION

It is well known that access to large patient populations and low cost are the major drivers of the move toward globalization of clinical trials. Despite globalization, however, slower-than-planned enrollment remains the norm for most clinical trials. Given the success of patient recruitment strategies in Western countries, it is reasonable to ask whether these same strategies might provide even better access to patients in emerging regions. This is not a trivial question, as cultural acceptability of various tactics commonly used in Western countries can be highly variable in other regions of the world. This book comprehensively addresses the recruitment of patients in a global environment, with a focus on both challenges encountered and solutions. Special interest chapters on recruiting patients in emerging regions for clinical trials such as Asia Pacific, Central and Eastern Europe and Latin America will serve as a great resource for sponsors and CROs planning trials in these areas.

A second major trend over the last few years has been the increased understanding that retaining patients in clinical trials is every bit as important as recruitment. As clinical trials with lengthy endpoints such as overall survival become more common, and as trials increasingly focus on drug safety, there is a great need to minimize patients who are lost to follow-up. Patient retention also is an important focus of regulatory agencies, and failure to retain patients can even invalidate the conclusions of a trial. This book treats recruitment and retention as "equal partners," with extensive coverage of this important topic throughout the book.

Despite the cost savings associated with the globalization of trials, the cost of conducting trials remains very high. Some costs, such as those associated with fulfilling GCP requirements, are essentially mandatory. Others, including funds spent on patient recruitment and retention, are discretionary and should be spent only if there is a defined (or at least reasonably expected) return on investment. For this reason, the clinical trials industry has begun to demand that providers of patient recruitment and retention services develop "metrics" showing that proposed strategies will result in a positive return on investment, either from direct reduction of the cost of conducting a trial or from accelerating its completion. This can, of course, be a challenging endeavor, as recruitment and retention tactics are rarely used in isolation. And for strategies such as social media that are newcomers on the patient recruitment and retention scene, there has been insufficient time to learn what is effective. Nevertheless, there is an appropriate demand on the part of clinical trial sponsors to measure the effectiveness of what we do, and if we are to remain relevant we need to rise to the challenge.

This valuable and timely book provides a comprehensive overview of the current "state of the art" in patient recruitment and retention. I know I speak for all readers in expressing my appreciation to Diana Anderson-Foster and all of the expert contributors for sharing their knowledge of this important area.

Martin Lee, M.D.
Executive Vice President, DAVA Oncology, LP

CHAPTER ONE

Mobilizing Strategy in a Global Environment

By Diana L. Anderson-Foster, Ph.D.

By conservative estimates, the global clinical research industry has experienced an 18% annual growth rate in recent years, spurred by lower labor costs, less competition and larger numbers of treatment-naïve patients in emerging markets. In December 2011, www.clinicaltrials.gov listed 21,430 open trials actively recruiting subjects, of which more than half were outside the United States. The typical late-stage clinical study—sponsored by small, mid-size and large companies—is now conducted in an average 34 countries, and in more than 70 countries on average for the top 20 sponsors.[1] The years 2003 through 2012 can be best characterized as a period of intense globalization and the emergence and growth of investigative sites based in more remote regions of the globe.[1]

This pattern picked up pace from 2005 to 2009, when the number of trials conducted in non-traditional (i.e., non-European and non-American) research countries more than doubled, from 21,653 in 2005 to 46,059 in 2009, per the European Medicines Agency (EMA).[2] In 2010, an impressive 78% of all subjects who participated in clinical trials were enrolled at non-U.S. sites, according to the Office of the Inspector General. Among those non-U.S. subjects, 58% were enrolled at sites in Western Europe and 26% were at sites in Central and South America. Of particular note, trials in Central and South America were an average 10 times larger than enrollments in Western Europe.[3]

Throughout this industry evolution, subject enrollment has remained the most confounding element in timely completion of global clinical trials, prompting drug and device manufacturers to spend $2.9 billion on patient recruitment services.[4] Yet getting patients to consent to research participation is but one step in the process. Keeping patients engaged through trial completion is vital to ensuring long-term trial success. It is, therefore, essential to mobilize strategies that minimize cost, maximize recruitment and avert subject attrition.

Figure 1: The evolution of patient recruitment

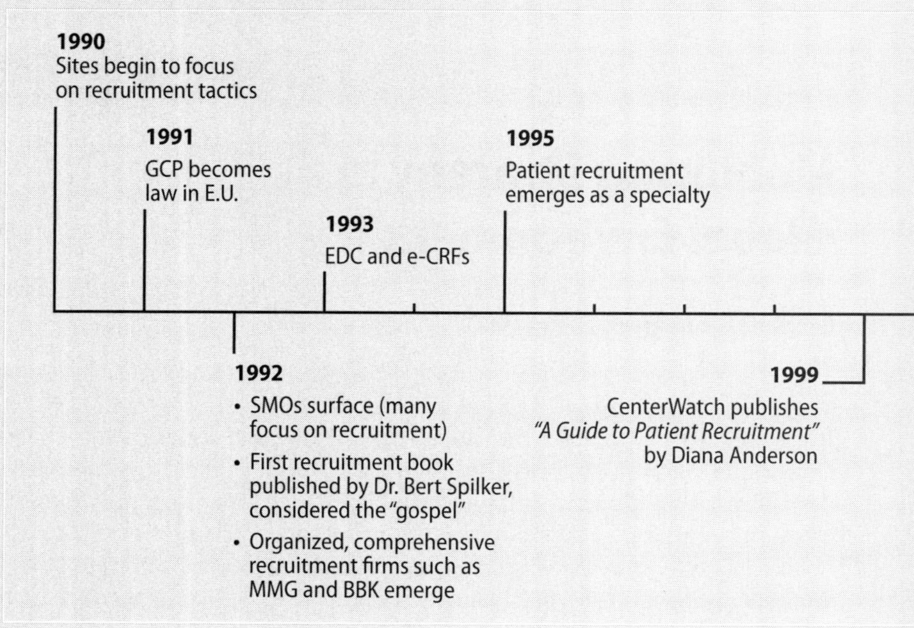

Patient Recruitment Professionals Gain Prominence

With the success of clinical trials so heavily contingent on reaching enrollment targets, sponsors are seeking service providers that offer patient recruitment as a core competency. Once a task largely relegated to site staff, patient recruitment has evolved from rudimentary methods to complex models requiring specialized expertise. To ensure the process runs smoothly, companies look for providers that possess superior metric reporting processes, program management capabilities, experience in the clinical area under study, operational problem-solving skills and global reach. This growing trend spawned the formation of the Patient Recruitment Organization Steering Committee, an ad hoc group of patient recruitment professionals whose mission is to improve the understanding, quality and effectiveness of clinical trial patient recruitment and retention services within the pharmaceutical, device and biotech industries.

As global clinical trials continue to hit historic highs, competition among Contract Research Organizations (CROs) and Patient Recruitment Organizations (PROs) has increased. Over the past decade, the five leading CROs have expanded their services to include patient recruitment. The CRO market is an estimated $24 billion, up from $14 billion in 2006, according to a report by Business Insights. Though large, the CRO space is highly fragmented, with more than 1,100 organizations worldwide despite consolidation. Conversely, there are about a dozen established PROs specializing in clinical trials and an ever-growing number of smaller, niche companies.

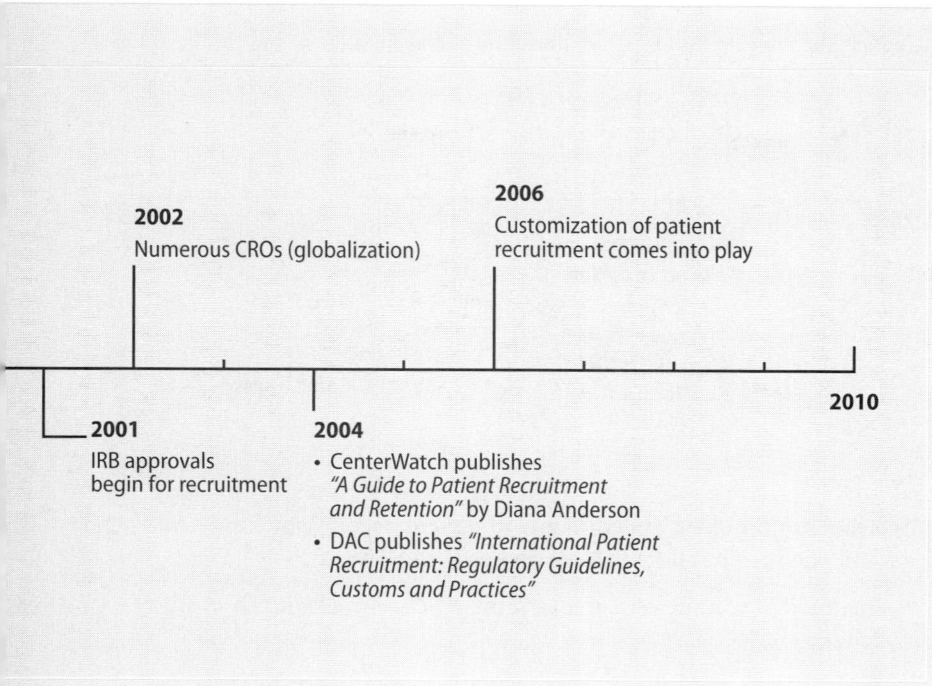

Securing Site Commitment

Achieving enrollment success also lies in clinical trial sponsors' understanding that patient recruitment and retention strategies are only as effective as the clinical sites commissioned to implement the plans. By aggressively educating and engaging sites, sponsors can mitigate competitive challenges, maintain statistical advantage and realize enrollment success. Central to this effort are identifying high-performing sites equipped to execute program plans, training clinical staff in recruitment fundamentals and motivating sites throughout enrollment. Yet, before any of these steps can occur, the trial sponsor must be fully educated about, invested in and committed to the strategy. After all, though there is shared responsibility for execution, the onus of outcome rests squarely with the sponsor as program progenitor and enforcer.

Securing site commitment to patient recruitment strategies requires gaining insights into sites' motivations and challenges. To that end, surveys were recently conducted among sites participating in 10 different clinical research studies across four continents and 37 countries.[5] Of 384 respondents, 58% were nurses and clinical research coordinators, and 42% were principal investigators. A striking 78.2% of participants reported their sites had failed to meet patient enrollment goals. This feedback aligns with a November 2010 *CenterWatch* report underscoring that half of all sites under-enroll or fail to enroll a single patient, while 30% of sites provide 70% of all evaluable subjects. Consequences for sites that perform poorly run the gamut up to and including closure.

Figure 2: The ongoing shift in patient recruitment players

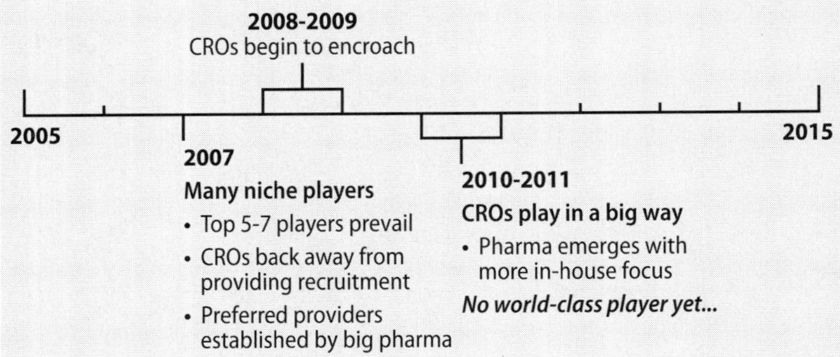

So what are the chief impediments to patient enrollment from a site perspective? The research noted above reveals the following:

- Insufficient volume of patients at the practice level who meet study criteria
- Lack of study awareness among potential referring physicians
- Absence of study awareness materials targeted to patients

Despite these challenges, some sites may fail to fully follow sponsor-approved patient recruitment programs. In regions where these strategies are permissible, less than half of survey respondents reported use of direct-to-patient advertising (45.5%) and slightly more than half participated in community outreach events (51.5%). Conversely, 73% expressed interest in recruitment materials such as brochures and posters, while 64.5% wanted support with physician mailings. Though the data may seem contradictory or counter-intuitive on the surface, it exposes the need for better site selection and recruitment-focused site training.

Site selection is, arguably, an arduous task that requires both operational and regulatory acumen. Though it may seem obvious, it cannot be overstated: The first consideration in selecting sites should be access to patients. To maximize access, prevalence data may be used to identify sites serving defined patient populations within a specific geographic area. Thorough analyses during pre-qualification visits will ensure sites are equipped to recruit patients, prepared for a regulatory audit and capable of protecting trial subjects.

Reinforcement Through Training

Once sites have been identified, the next critical determinant for hitting enrollment targets is to obtain maximum program buy-in and understanding among investigators and staff. One strategy to achieve this is a Best Practices webinar series. For example, 63% of global diabetes sites surveyed ranked webinars as an effective recruitment strategy. Attended by investigators and clinical research coordinators at all participating sites, webinars promote personal accountability for screening activity and allow sites to discuss challenges and strategize solutions. Sponsors can maximize webinar participation by offering multiple sessions with at least two date and time options.

Subsequent sessions should cover the rudiments of effective patient recruitment. Sponsors today are more progressive in understanding the value of training investigative sites in patient enrollment strategies, and many invest resources accordingly. Some sites provide training for study coordinators through certification programs offered by the Association of Clinical Research Professionals (ACRP) and the Society of Clinical Research Association (SOCRA). While these programs have utility, they largely focus on the principles of Good Clinical Practice, not the specifics of patient recruitment, and they do not have global application.

Sponsors should evaluate sites and plot a training strategy that will have the greatest impact. The training medium will depend on what needs to be conveyed and the audience's level of experience. Self-paced computer training may be effective for content that is self-explanatory, while interactive programs may be more useful for other situations. Teleconferencing can also be productive.

In addition, sponsors can augment the enrollment effort by hiring patient recruitment specialists who offer training as a core service. The benefits of such training are evident and enduring. Training improves processes, boosts performance, reduces turnover and raises morale. For example, one sponsor reported a 22% increase in enrollment activity within three months of recruitment-focused site training. Moreover, sponsor-funded training engenders site trust and allegiance. Consequently, when presented with the opportunity to participate in competing studies, sites often favor sponsors who have demonstrated a commitment to their professional development by investing in their training. In becoming a "sponsor of choice," a company may increase its access to high-performing, highly trained sites.

Recruitment Strategies

Although access to potential patients in some world regions is apparent, low levels of awareness and interest in participating in clinical trials, coupled with negative perceptions and skepticism, may hinder recruitment in some countries. Understanding cross-cultural recruitment practices poses challenges for sponsors and CROs. Some sponsors have limited experience with formal patient recruitment programs, let alone the ability to grasp how to leverage patient recruitment support for a global trial. Furthermore, few patient recruitment service providers have experience managing multinational recruitment campaigns. The regulatory and ethical climates relating to recruitment practices vary widely, and dissecting the regulations and guidelines pertaining to patient recruitment can be daunting. Every country has a history, experience and research culture that demands a customized approach to recruitment.

A multidimensional patient recruitment strategy is required to compete globally amid changing industry dynamics. A program's viability is determined by its ability to captivate and inform the target audience, meet regulatory standards governing patient communication and allow for accurate tracking, monitoring and metrics reporting. Global recruitment programs must be developed with an understanding that external initiatives may be less relevant or appropriate in densely populated regions with specialized healthcare institutions than in other areas, where patient access is more restrictive due to geographic spread or competing trials. For these regions, tools and materials developed to facilitate patient identification within individual institutions are more appropriate than public awareness-building campaigns. For example, U.S. strategies often include social media and direct-to-patient advertising, whereas ROW initiatives emphasize physician education and site support.

The trial sponsor has the authority to require patient recruitment plan compliance among clinical sites. In some cases, sponsors allow sites to select strategies from the plan at their own discretion. If this is the case, measures must be established that define how and where initiatives will be deployed. Additionally, sponsors should establish written policies pertaining to patient recruitment strategy noncompliance.

Maintaining Momentum and Motivation

Frequent communication is essential to keeping sites informed and engaged throughout a clinical trial. There are various tools to support this effort, including site newsletters, electronic communication, study web sites with site pages and even study-branded support items that promote study awareness. Within the site schematic, the clinical research coordinator indisputably holds one of the most vital positions in the context of patient access. Working in tandem with principal investigators, coordinators are responsible for screening eligible patients and establishing a positive rapport with them, as well as recording accurate and timely data, reporting adverse events promptly to the sponsor and ensuring safety for all research participants.

Having a supportive trial sponsor can alleviate the day-to-day pressures clinical teams experience. Establish a positive rapport with sites before a study is initiated. Additionally, encouraging camaraderie and cooperation within each site is a strategic move.

In the busy field of clinical research, it's easy to neglect the people who devote their time to participate. Companies can solve this by recognizing top performance and dedication among clinical teams. This can be done in the site newsletter, during a web conference or via other venues. Simple acknowledgment and affirmation go a long way in boosting morale—and performance.

A number of variables contribute to the success of a clinical trial. Among these are the establishment of rapport, trust and mutual commitment to study goals among research sites, the CRO and the sponsor. From these relationships comes enthusiasm among sites to embrace and execute recruitment strategies. Taking the time to invest in relationships may be the best recruitment strategy of all.

In any competitive environment, achievers understand how to leverage their abilities to meet the most pressing needs of customers. As the industry matures, sponsors have become acutely aware that successful patient recruitment requires more than mining patient databases and placing occasional advertisements. The process demands professional organizations with strategic foresight, therapeutic expertise and operational acumen that can deliver evidence-based results, i.e., metrics. Tactics for squaring off with market competitors originate at the point of hire by building teams with the acumen and attitude to interface with the industry's customer base. Today's patient recruitment organizations are defining the future of clinical trials—building recruitment programs from the ground up, coaching sites to meet program benchmarks, monitoring outcomes and delivering return on investment.

Author Biography

Over a career spanning more than 25 years, Diana L. Anderson-Foster, Ph.D., has helped pioneer best practices in patient recruitment and retention for global clinical trials—first as founder, president and CEO of D. Anderson & Company and today as president of DAC Patient Recruitment Services. Her book credits include *International Patient Recruitment: Regulatory Guidelines, Customs and Practices; A Guide to Patient Recruitment; and A Guide to Patient Recruitment and Retention.* In 2006, PharmaVOICE named her among the 100 Most Inspiring People in the Life Sciences Industry. She also received an International Women of Influence Award from the Global EXEC Women's International Council in 2008, among other honors.

References

1. Getz K.A., Zuckerman R. *Today's global site landscape.* Applied Clinical Trials. 2010 June: 34-38. Available from: http://appliedclinicaltrials online.findpharma.com

2. SOMO (Centre for Research on Multinational Corporations). *Putting contract research organisations on the radar.* Amsterdam: SOMO, February 2011. Available from: http://somo.nl

3. Office of Inspector General, HHS. *Challenges to FDA's ability to monitor and inspect foreign clinical trials* (OEI-01-08-00510). OIG, June 2010. Available from: http://oig.hhs.gov/oei/reports/oei-01-08-00510.pdf

4. Mintz, Cliff. *Social Media's Impact on Clinical Trial Enrollment.* Life Science Leader. November 2010

5. DAC Patient Recruitment Services, Global Diabetes Study

CHAPTER TWO

Operational Challenges and Solutions in Recruitment Implementation Around the World

By Bonnie A. Brescia

Introduction

In years past, adding countries to a randomized clinical trial was often a last-minute solution to enhance patient enrollment and complete trials. Today, executing multinational clinical trials is a requirement for companies invested in drug development. As such, patient recruitment is no longer a second thought but a crucial process in clinical trial planning and execution.

A key driver for this trend is drug and biologic manufacturers' continued market expansion, as they seek to make compounds available worldwide. While the United States is still the largest pharmaceutical market in the world, other regions show much stronger growth. China was predicted to grow 25–27% to more than $50 billion in 2011 and surpass Japan as the second-largest market as early as 2020.[1]

The potential for cost savings also drives the inclusion of developing countries in global trials; however, adding countries increases the complexity of operational and infrastructure management. With innumerable individuals and entities to be managed, the onus is on global study managers to oversee multiple countries, including those with which they may be unfamiliar. The team lead also must deal with prolific regulatory requirements, while paying attention to cultural differences in business conduct and communications and keeping stakeholders' attention focused on the goal of study completion.

In response to these market demands over the last decade, patient recruitment has evolved into a robust and refined discipline. When sophisticated offerings migrate from Western countries to emerging clinical trial markets, they contribute to the development of advanced research infrastructure in these countries. And as the industry recognizes the importance of fostering partnerships among the many parties involved in research—clinicians, scientists, research sites and patients—this infrastructure becomes a critical factor in successful study implementation.

Implementing the most current patient recruitment practices allows global team leaders to streamline trial functions. By investing in methodologies that integrate age-old knowledge of human relationships with recent innovations and technologies, the clinical trial industry can bring improved healthcare solutions to the public much faster.

Clinical teams look to the evolution of patient recruitment for the "silver bullet" of study enrollment—the perfect recruitment tool to attract patients, engage sites and ensure on-time completion of their trial. New and exciting recruitment techniques blossom alongside global advances in telecommunications and internet connectivity, providing the opportunity to leverage these new resources for clinical trial enrollment.

This chapter highlights some of these new tools, then re-focuses on the nitty-gritty of patient recruitment—the integration of recruitment principles into clinical trial planning and implementation. When recruitment begins with the basic building blocks of good strategies and planning, global study teams can launch successful outreach and enrollment efforts using new as well as tried-and-true techniques.

New Trends

The field of patient recruitment advances on an almost daily basis. Recent innovations point to the ascending importance of collaboration and cooperation between clinical research sponsors and their partners in execution and between patients and the clinical trial enterprise. The ever-expanding technological channels for communication and connection facilitate these collaborations and provide the opportunity to strengthen the relationships between these key stakeholders.

A Franchise Approach to Patient Recruitment

Forward-thinking sponsors of clinical research maximize their resources by coordinating recruitment efforts not just across one protocol and many countries, but across many protocols in a single therapeutic area for one or many countries. Drug developers have a long history of strategizing compound development and they are now applying such thinking to planning and implementing the clinical trial process.

Financial drivers for this trend include the pressure of economic globalization as many countries experience economic downturns. Clinical research companies tackle this issue by finding ways for clinical teams to work closely with procurement and contracting to add value and reduce expenses through combined efforts for multiple related trials. Joint planning and execution increases cost savings and reduces duplication of efforts. For example, pooling budgets and other resources to conduct outreach and communication campaigns for multiple studies results in less expenditure to generate more potential patients at investigative sites.

Global clinical trials

Large, global, commercial clinical trials show increased growth:

- The number of clinical trials (phases I-III) worldwide has risen from 40,000 in 2000 to 59,000 in 2006.[2]
- In 2008, 80% of U.S.-approved marketing applications for drugs and biologics contained data from foreign clinical trials and over half of clinical trial subjects and sites were located outside the U.S.[3]
- In addition, the frequency of foreign-based studies, as evidenced by FDA 1572 forms, has increased from 16.3% (in 2001) to 35.5% (in 2007) of all studies.[4]

Cost savings for global trials can be significant, but not across the board:

- A 2006 assessment of global clinical trial costs showed that in comparison to the U.S., the least expensive venue for a trial was Russia, at 40% of the cost, with China at 52% and India at 56% of U.S. costs.[5]
- The cost of recruiting a patient in Japan is nearly 2.5 times as high as in the U.S.[6]

Figure 1: Overall indexed clinical trial costs

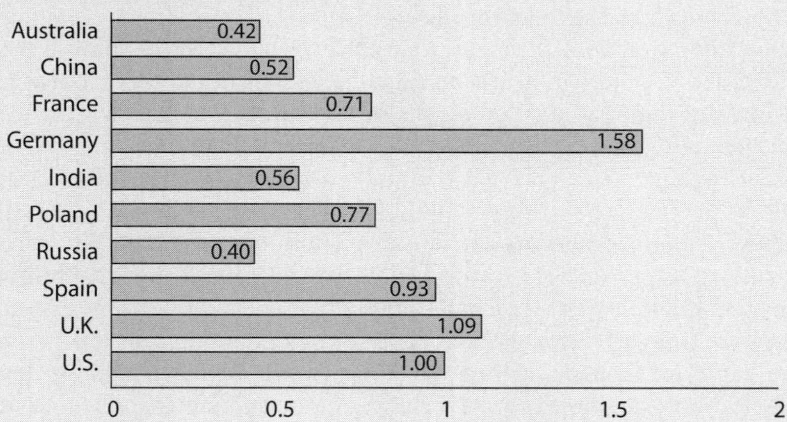

Source: FastTrack Systems Global Cost Databases, 2005-2006

Figure 2: Global costs of patient recruitment

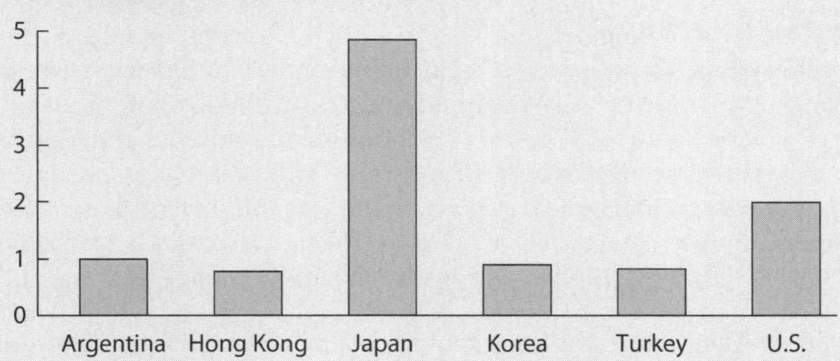

Source: Indiana University Center for Bioethics

The challenges of expanding operations across multiple protocols include breaking open the traditional silo model of "one protocol, one clinical team." The franchise approach requires clinical team leaders to work across lines, share knowledge and be open to new perspectives, which initially seems like extra work. Senior management can support cross-team communication by building and giving access to central databases of collective knowledge gained and by encouraging all to make adjustments to clinical operations, financial and procurement processes.

Going Mobile

The clinical research enterprise must consider and incorporate the communication and connection methods of today to continue to attract and retain clinical trial participants. The internet, mobile technologies and social networks such as Facebook and its international equivalents—Mixi in Japan or Renren in the People's Republic of China—increasingly connect people around the world. For patients, there are various health web sites that gather and share information and experiences on a daily and even minute-by-minute basis.

As patients increase their knowledge, they engage in more questioning of and collaboration with their physicians. When involved with clinical trials, patients expect shared information from the investigator and site staff as well as from the company developing the new treatment. In global patient recruitment efforts, the following digital aids increasingly facilitate this flow of information:

Mobile Devices—Healthcare consumers around the world are likely to have more access to personal electronic devices than an average study coordinator managing multiple trials via email, data entry and spreadsheets on a desktop computer. Study participants expect appointment reminders by text messages and apps for their smartphones to enter patient-reported data. By developing technologies on platforms including mobile phones, handheld devices and computer tablets, patient recruitment specialists help clinical research staff keep pace with the increasingly savvy healthcare consumer.

Social Media—Finding patients for a trial often means finding them where they live—a media perspective. Today that includes not just television and radio, but the world of social media. Market research tools allow sponsors to target, observe and record activity on social media outlets to better understand the patients they seek to enroll into trials. This information can be used to shape messages and campaigns to communicate with potential candidates. In many countries, outreach through social media advertising is a viable way to convey study opportunities and attract patients to trials.

Patient-Driven, Online Communities—In the dynamic environment of online patient communities, people exchange, share and publish health information to benefit one another and their wider communities. These portals should also be recognized as potential platforms for patient participation and collaboration in the scientific endeavor of clinical research. There are many methods for sponsors to communicate and interact with online patient communities, conveying information, generating interest and building relationships around clinical trial opportunities.

Electronic Medical Record Systems—Though EMRs have yet to meet the expectations of matching patients to protocol requirements, recent developments in the technology show potential. As EMR systems rapidly gain market penetration and refine their data normalization and search functioning, new web-based cloud computing models replace the installed systems of the early players in the EMR market. The best systems are able to transform open text into redefined and searchable data for analysis to support clinical research.

No matter the sophistication of a country's technology, patients around the world share the basic desire to improve their health, understand their options and maintain communication with their support networks, including peers and physicians. Understanding and maximizing new technologies is a very important stepping stone for clinical researchers seeking to connect with patients.

Recruitment Processes as Integral to Trial Planning

Patient recruitment goes beyond providing sites with recruitment tools, no matter how "new and shiny." Rather, it's a systematic and comprehensive approach best integrated into every level of clinical trial planning and execution—from the early development of a protocol through study completion.

Even for those who feel they "know" recruitment techniques, there's far more to actual success than being aware of or even familiar with the tools. The skill to analyze data from many sources, apply a recruitment lens to the data and practice hands-on application serves to truly cement knowledge and capability.

Feasibility

Including patient recruitment data and perspectives enhances global clinical trial feasibility. Follow this 5-point guide to be sure your efforts benefit from enrollment-focused analysis:

Five-Point Guide to Patient Recruitment Feasibility

1. **Analyze your protocol based on recruitment-related aspects.** This means collecting information from many sources, assessing each factor for a positive or negative impact on recruitment and weighting the factors in importance. This results in an overall analysis of the ease or difficulty of recruiting for the trial.

Primary Enrollment Principle (PEP)

The PEP is designed for a quick check of enrollment success, especially for studies with a broad potential pool of patients and few protocol limitations.

e = (r * t * s) + n

Where:

e – randomized patients

r – randomization rate (patients/site/month)

t – enrollment period (months)

s – number of sites actively randomizing patients

n – number of patients already randomized

If you have four of the five variables, you can solve for the last one. For example:

150 patients needed

12-month enrollment period

20 investigative sites

No patients are currently randomized

Solve for '**r**'

e = (**r** x **t** x **s**) + **n**

150 = (**r** x 12 x 20) + 0

150/240 = **r** = 0.625 patients/site/month

Take care to develop this projection for each country involved in the study. In France, sites may be active for eight recruitment months; in Brazil four months; in China two months. This variability could shift the average enrollment rate from .625 to nearly 2.0 patients/site/month, resulting in an extremely different feasibility.

2. **Use mathematical formulas to make general assessments of enrollment feasibility** based on the number of countries and sites, time allotted for enrollment and patients already enrolled (if the trial has started). One example is the Primary Enrollment Principle (see sidebar).

3. **Use referral funnels** to gain a more accurate gauge of eligible patients at sites. Rather than rely solely on feasibility estimates based on general knowledge and guestimates, it is possible to apply the inclusion/exclusion criteria and other factors to determine a more realistic number of patients that might become randomized.

4. **Compare your assessment data** from these methods to the feasibility estimates from countries and sites. If discrepancies appear, make adjustments to allocations or determine the need for support/intervention to reach designated deadlines.

5. **Create enrollment projection models.** Using the data analysis described above, clinical leads can develop templates for "running the numbers" for anticipated screening and randomization. The model is useful before the study starts, and once under way, can run current data to show projected end points, alerting teams before potential problems become crises.

Country Selection

Assessing countries from a patient recruitment perspective turns up some surprising insights. What might seem an advantage—ready access to medical care—might actually be a negative if patients don't see clinical trials as an attractive alternative. Factors that seem negative, such as an over-diagnosed or treated condition, can be overcome with proper identification and advanced planning. Investing in a comprehensive assessment of countries based on a variety of factors provides global study teams with the data and results to inform selection and support of countries for the trial. Recruitment-related factors should be identified for each protocol and then weighted in importance for likely enrollment impact.

Site Selection

As with country selection, modified site selection processes that include patient recruitment-specific variables allow a global study team to study factors that were not considered consistently in the past. Site reporting and past experience provide good general indicators but may not accurately predict enrollment for an upcoming trial, no matter the similarity to previous studies. Some general recruitment-related factors to be assessed include: staffing capacity, knowledge/motivation to enroll protocol, communication skills with patients, equipment/facilities, contracting/budgeting and regulatory speed. Again, the full power of this methodology lies in comparing sites to one another using a study-specific, yet uniform, set of measures. This allows clinical trial leaders to rate and rank sites for likely levels of performance, giving a more rational basis for selection or exclusion of a given research site.

Recruitment/Retention Strategies

Recruitment strategies start with good planning and rely on the development of country and site recruitment plans. Tools and techniques support the plans—from the now-standard range of materials to the evolving skills in coaching, collaborating and supporting investigators and site staff. Armed with knowledge of the protocol's strengths and weaknesses for recruitment, as well as the main motivating factors for patients to enroll, global study teams empower themselves and their sites to make recruitment plans and use recruitment tools. In addition, study monitors can focus their efforts to help sites with the key recruitment touch points: identifying, consenting,

Figure 3: Recruitment funnel worksheet for HIV study

Total number of patients expected to be screened	12 patients
Expected screen fail percentage	50%
Randomization goal for the site	6 patients
Enrollment period (number of active months from FPI to LPI)	12 months
Required screening rate	1.0 patient/site/month
Required randomization rate	0.5 patient/site/month
Key enrollment variable	**Enter number of patients**
1. Total number of patients currently diagnosed with HIV at the principal investigator's site.	
2. Of the patients entered above, please estimate the total number of patients who have not yet received treatment for their HIV (treatment-naive patients).	
3. Of the patients you entered above in row 2, please estimate the total number of patients who do not have chronic Hepatitis B.	
4. Of the patients you entered above in row 3, please estimate the total number of patients who are not participating in other clinical trials.	
(Add any further I/E criteria that may affect the number of available patients at the site.)	
5. Of the patients you entered above in row 4, how many will the investigator approach and discuss study participation with? (i.e., total number of patients approached about study participation.)	
6. Of the patients you entered above in row 5, how many will be interested in and consent to study participation? (i.e., total number of patients consented into study.) This is the total number of patients that can be screened.	
7. Based on the screen-fail rate of 50%, how many of the consented patients that you entered in row 6 will randomize?	

Source: BBK Worldwide

Figure 4: Analysis of recruitment barriers

Even though Italy and Russia fall into the "poor enrollment" category, they should not necessarily be excluded from the study. However, you may need to increase recruitment support or reduce enrollment targets.

Key variable	Nat'l health system	Gov't/reg. issues	Treatment algorithm	Recruitment process	Disease prevalence	Access to care	Weighted score	Recruitment status
Weighting	20%	15%	15%	10%	30%	10%	100%	
U.S.	1	1	1	0	1	-1	0.70	Good
Germany	0	1	1	0	1	0	0.60	
Australia	0	0	1	0	1	1	0.55	
U.K.	0	0	1	0	1	1	0.55	
Argentina	0	0	1	-1	0	1	0.15	Average
Finland	0	0	0	1	0	0	0.10	
Austria	0	0	1	0	-1	1	-0.05	
Italy	-1	-1	-1	-1	0	1	-0.50	Poor
Russia	-1	-1	-1	0	-1	1	-0.70	

Source: BBK Worldwide, 2009

Monitoring Site Enrollment Performance and Reallocating Resources Where Needed

Recruitment plans, along with a good method for tracking real-time recruitment data, are indispensible for ongoing tracking and assessment of site performance. Both give country leads and monitors/clinical research associates (CRAs) a way to spot weaknesses and offer support to sites needing to raise recruitment rates. With knowledge and tools, they can tackle potential barriers *before* they arise. New technologies allow the tracking of study data through a recruitment filter, drawing the metrics into reports that allow easy analysis of where sites are struggling. With this kind of monitoring, proactive clinical trial leaders take steps to address anticipated shortfalls in screening, consent, randomization or retention/compliance.

Site Perspectives

At a global level, site concerns remain consistent across countries—they value their relationships with sponsors. To develop strong relationships with their sites, sponsors must thoroughly understand their needs and consider

Figure 5: Patient recruitment touch points and recruitment tools that support them

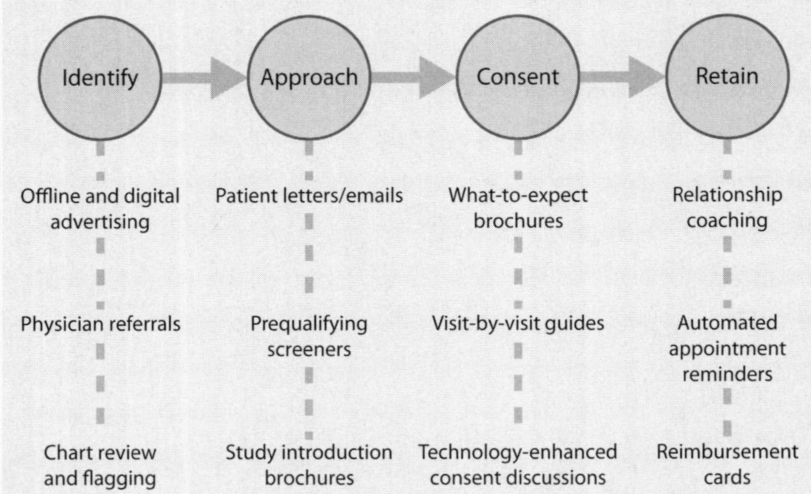

Source: BBK Worldwide

ways to customize support by country and by site wherever possible. This plays out in several significant aspects, including the fulfillment of the contract in terms of enrollment compensation, the consistency of contact with study representatives and the support of sites in managing difficult-to-enroll studies.

Sites as a Recruitment and Retention Audience

While CRAs often are closest to the details of relationships with sites, from contract and budgeting to regulatory approvals, from monitoring data to working on recruitment strategies, all levels of clinical trial leaders can benefit from understanding and incorporating site perspectives.

Analyzing a protocol from the perspective of a site reveals the strengths and challenges for 1) recruiting the site for the study and 2) knowing where sites will need help enrolling patients. The same process can be applied to retention by 1) asking where the challenges lie for keeping a site motivated and enthusiastic and 2) anticipating potential participant retention or compliance gaps.

What Sponsors Can Offer

A good relationship must be founded on clear expectations from both sides. Sponsors can apply this to the contracting and budgeting process, particularly in the area of compensation. In the early phases of trial planning, sponsors have expected sites to provide feasibility estimates as part of the selection process. The entire clinical research enterprise acknowledges that this method results in less-than-optimal accurate projections. Some CROs and sponsors now offer sites a stipend for feasibility assessments to ensure better quality and equity in the selection process. The same careful attention is important to sites once a trial starts, with emphasis on timely payments and reimbursements. When sponsors stay attuned to site needs, they positively affect motivation to enroll patients.

Establishing and monitoring recruitment plans allow CRAs to identify issues before they become a crisis and proactively step in to assist sites. Ideally, the sponsor will build in the potential for customizing site support on a country or individual site level. This may take the form of culturally adapted materials, different combinations of tools for different sites or training for CRAs on specific site barriers to empower them to better coach sites. For sponsors, determining the point at which a site's contract should be terminated for non-performance—and communicating performance expectations to the site—helps when such decisions must be made.

Investigative sites consistently report they most value the opportunity to work with the same monitor for all studies sponsored by one company or staffed by one CRO. While sites recognize this isn't always possible, it reinforces the importance of relationships in every aspect of clinical trial operations. Secondly, sites want to be respected as scientific and business partners: told the entire story and paid fairly and on time.

Patient Perspectives

Those who conduct clinical research tend to focus on the operational, medical and logistical aspects of the project, for good reasons. However, we must increase awareness among sponsors and the general public about the importance of the patient's role in bringing new treatments to market.

Polls of patients in the U.S. and Europe show a consistent pattern over the last 10 years—people around the world recognize the importance of clinical research in developing new medical treatments and are willing to do their part if they are provided the opportunity and education to make informed decisions. While patients in Western countries have long taken a more proactive approach to their healthcare, those in emerging clinical trial markets increasingly seek new sources of information in addition to their physicians. The internet and new mobile technologies make information much more accessible, and the rise of online communities attracts patients from many countries who wish to share their health information and experiences.

Education/Informed Decision Making

The moment a patient decides to participate in a trial is a critical point—it could mean the difference between an evaluable patient and a dropout. When done well, the informed consent/decision-making process provides

Patient attitudes toward clinical trials

- Over 80% of Americans and 68% of Europeans would consider participating in a clinical trial, but only 13% of Americans and 5% of Europeans have been given the opportunity.[7]
- CenterWatch reports that 94 percent of people recognize the importance of participating in clinical research to assist in the advancement of medical science.
- Nearly 75% of the general public states they have little to no knowledge about the clinical research enterprise and the participation process, according to The Center for Information and Study on Clinical Research Participation (CISCRP).
- Only a small percentage of Americans have participated in a trial—a consistent 3% to 7% of the population—but of these, over 80% say they would do it again,[8] indicating the experience generally seems to be positive.

patients with a clear picture of what it takes to qualify for the study and what will be required once they enroll. When patients fully understand the extent of the time commitment, visit schedule, tests and medication requirements, compensation and risks/benefits, they become much more likely to stay engaged until study completion. Investing this time up front pays off later, especially for longer trials with higher attrition risks.

A good relationship between the patient and site is critical to study compliance and retention. When site staff focus on communicating with patients during and between appointments and helping them through actual or potential difficulties, this fosters good will among patients.

Partnership

In any partnership, both parties take on potential risks for potential benefits. Sponsors of research and their representatives, from CROs to sites, take on financial and operational risks for the potential benefit of bringing new medications to the public. Patients who participate are likewise taking on health risks for the hope of potential gains, either for themselves or for future patients with their diseases or conditions.

Contemporary patient recruitment methods take the patient perspective into account when assessing the impact of the protocol on patient motivations, selecting countries and sites and providing strategies and tools to support informed consent and commitment to the study. It is important to separate the patient viewpoint from those of the clinical team, the CRO and other vendors, the CRAs and even the sites. All of these audiences may project their own ideas about patient participation onto the population. Teams that step back and assess the realities of patients and their motivations to participate contribute immeasurably to recruitment and retention success.

Getting to know patients

To develop a relationship, there must be give and take. Consider these questions from a patient's point of view—the answers influence his or her attitude and feelings about participating in a trial:

- Do you talk about your condition/disease often? With whom?
- If you could get one thing from your physician, what would it be?
- What aspect of your condition/disease is particularly hard to live with?
- How is your condition/disease perceived by the general public? By the medical community?
- If there were a clinical trial for your condition, what would you want it to explore?

Expanding Recruitment Tools and Techniques

The status of regulatory acceptance of patient recruitment tools and techniques varies around the world. Research shows, however, that where such methods enhance patient information and understanding of clinical research, they receive legal and ethical support. Very few countries' legislation mentions, much less prohibits, communication outreach to patients about clinical trials.[9] Surveys of ethics committees around the world reveal the acceptability of using a wide range of printed and broadcast materials to educate patients.[10]

The question is not "What tools can be used in what country?," but "How can we best communicate the study opportunity to patients?" The answer guides the types of materials and advertising needed to attract patients, and if the messages and methods are reasonable, ethics committees will be very open to considering almost any tool. The bottom line: will the tool benefit the patient's awareness and understanding of this study and/or the site's ability to communicate with patients and other physicians?

Given the wide range of site and monitor attitudes toward and acceptance of recruitment materials, assuming a positive approach has no down side. With all materials submitted to ethics committees, approval offers the potential for using these materials to fill recruitment gaps, should they arise.

Managing Costs

When global teams plan for recruitment early in the global trial process, they build resources into the budget to develop materials that can be adapted by each country. The goal is to achieve a balance between cost/time efficiencies and customization of materials by country or even site.

Knowledge of regulatory speed for approvals and cultural acceptance of outreach items facilitate effective budget allocation decisions. Many companies follow a standard approach to developing recruitment materials for ethics review and approval, and then to holding them for production depending

Figure 6: Top 10 multinational recruitment tools for patients

1. Pamphlet explaining the study
2. Study visit guide detailing what happens at every visit
3. Poster
4. Patient letter
5. Advertising via traditional media
6. Online media and social networking
7. Web site with online screener
8. SMS text messaging
9. Retention items—thank you/appreciation cards, reimbursement cards, items of nominal value but related to helping with disease/condition
10. Relationships, relationships, relationships

Source: BBK Worldwide, data on file 2006-2011

on later need. In today's digital world, materials can be printed on demand at low cost.

Ethics Committees may not be the Limiting Factor

Surprisingly to some, the limiting attitudes toward the use of communication materials exist more among clinical team members such as country managers, CRA leaders, CRAs and sites than among ethics committee representatives. Basing their opinions on previous experience with other trials or governmental and ethics perspectives, sponsor and CRA staff sometimes assume certain recruitment tools and techniques will not be approved.

But as financial professionals warn, past experience does not necessarily predict the future. Both patients *and* ethics committees have shown increasing openness to receiving information about clinical trials that supports making informed decisions about participation. As the landscape in which people make healthcare decisions shifts, the clinical research industry must remain open to new possibilities and avenues for communicating with constituents.

Using Data to Guide Optimal Site Performance

Clinical trials rely heavily on technology for many aspects—planning, administration and collection of clinical data, analysis and reporting. There are countless systems available—some built in-house, some commercial—in-

Figure 7: Top 10 study enrollment and implementation aids for investigators worldwide

1. Speedy submission of recruitment tools to ethics committees
2. Inclusion/exclusion card
3. Study-visit guide detailing procedures by visit
4. Monitors with expertise in the disease and mastery of the protocol
5. Access to advertising budgets and resources
6. Access to and relationships with recruitment-knowledgable study representatives
7. Referring physician letter
8. Reasonable screen-fail projections and compensation
9. Appointment reminder services and tools
10. Relationships, relationships, relationships

Source: BBK Worldwide, data on file 2006-2011

cluding clinical trial management (CTM), clinical data management (CDM), electronic data collection (EDC), interactive voice response (IVR), patient reporting devices and more. Especially on a global level, consolidating and analyzing data across all sites and countries is crucial to managing time and costs, as well as to communicating progress throughout the organization.

While these technologies represent a vast improvement over the dated method of paper-based trials, they are only as valuable as the questions asked and data aggregated. Over the last 10 years, patient recruitment experts have recognized the need and developed technological solutions to specifically address enrollment questions. While CTM, EDC and IVR systems contain data points that relate to recruitment performance, they focus on different purposes and may not allow access to the most immediate, real-time data on enrollment processes. Thus emerged the era of patient recruitment management systems (PRMS), which draw on data from all sources, wherever the most immediate metrics are, to consolidate and report on recruitment and retention questions including:

- Are sites ahead of or behind schedule for screening numbers and rates?
- What are current randomization numbers and rates?
- How likely is the site to meet randomization rates based on screening rates?
- Where are the discrepancies in expectation versus performance?
- What are the points at which patients are dropping out? Are they patient- or site-related?

With this data, study leaders can create ongoing projection reports per site and per country that give a window into actual operations and help pinpoint problem areas sooner than later.

Because any plan is subject to change, contingency measures must be in place for recruitment efforts. These contingencies come into play only if actual enrollment numbers do not match projected numbers. By determining such triggers up front, shortfalls are linked to specific actions. For example, given the link between screening and randomization rates, tracking the often overlooked screening rates provides insight to site performance and likely ability to randomize. Establishing a date from the point of a site's initiation to its first screened patient provides CRAs with a good indicator for taking action, should sites miss the mark.

Conclusion

Multinational clinical trials, with all their attendant complexities and incredible contributions to science and medical advancement, are here to stay. Sponsors need to invest in their operational infrastructure to plan and run them well, including the crucial process of recruiting patients. With one eye on the big picture, drug development leaders must focus equal attention on the details of planning and execution to coordinate the profusion of parties involved in one global trial. Sponsors most likely to succeed in this endeavor will be process-oriented, nimble in making adjustments to plans when recruitment shows gaps and willing to invest significant funds up front rather than wait for a crisis.

Author Biography

Bonnie A. Brescia is co-founder of BBK Worldwide, a leader in patient recruitment for clinical research and development. A pioneer of patient recruitment over the last 28 years, Bonnie helped to shape the discipline and continues to be a well-recognized and highly sought after thought leader in the field. Her insights into the workings of the clinical research community inform BBK's product development, campaign execution and global expansion. Bonnie serves on the boards for The Center for Information and Study on Clinical Research Participation (CISCRP), Groundswell International, the Charles River School and the Advisory Committee at the University of Medicine and Dentistry of New Jersey (UMDNJ) masters in clinical research program. She is a guest lecturer at UMDNJ and Emerson College/Tufts University School of Medicine graduate program in health communications. In 2005, Bonnie was recognized by *PharmaVOICE* as one of the 100 most inspiring people in the industry. She is a graduate of Emerson College and received the Distinguished Alumni Award in 2011.

References

1. Business Insider, *CITI: Good News For Drug Makers, The Chinese Pharmaceutical Market Will Reach $200 Billion by 2020*, March 7, 2011, www.businessinsider.com
2. Clinicaltrials.gov.
3. Department of Health and Human Services, Office of Inspector General, *Challenges to FDA's Ability to Monitor and Inspect Foreign Clinical Trials*, June 2010.
4. "CenterWatch. State of the clinical trials industry: a sourcebook of charts and statistics. Boston: CenterWatch, 2009."p. 488.
5. FastTrack Systems Global Cost Databases, 2005–2006.
6. Presentation by Dr. Uden at 3rd Kitasato-Harvard Symposium, 2002
7. BBK Worldwide, Will & Why Survey, 2001, European Will & Why Survey, 2004
8. Ibid.
9. *International Patient Recruitment Regulatory Guidelines, Customs and Practices*, Diana L. Anderson, 2007
10. *Global Regulatory Attitudes Toward Communicating Directly with Patients: The Ethics Committee Survey: Results and Analysis*, BBK Worldwide, May 2005

CHAPTER THREE

Site Feasibility and Protocol Evaluation and the Relationship to Recruitment

By Beth Harper

The triumvirate of clinical trial success consists of an executable protocol, a group of capable and interested investigative sites and a qualified and motivated patient population. What sounds simple and straightforward is, in fact, extremely challenging and difficult to achieve. In this chapter we will explore the complexities and nuances that affect successful clinical trial participation. We will investigate the traditional approach to protocol evaluation and site feasibility assessment, along with associated results. We will examine why the traditional process fails to yield timely and predictable enrollment success and the root issues driving this failure. Finally, we will consider what it takes to ensure a good fit among the protocol, the sites and the patient population, and we will describe new approaches with the potential to produce more predictive and improved results.

While this chapter focuses on the process used with industry-sponsored clinical trials, many of the principles and recommendations discussed apply to all types of clinical trials (investigator initiated, foundation and government funded trials, etc.).

Factors Affecting Successful Clinical Trial Participation

From a patient recruitment and retention standpoint, a multitude of factors influence a subject's willingness and ability to join and stay in a clinical trial. These factors can generally be lumped into four key categories: protocol related, sponsor or CRO related, investigative site related and subject-related issues. Figure 1 illustrates many of the common factors that influence successful trial participation.

Adding to the complexity of the clinical trial process is the fact that each individual subject (and his or her family or caregiver) has different needs,

Figure 1: Factors that affect successful clinical trial participation

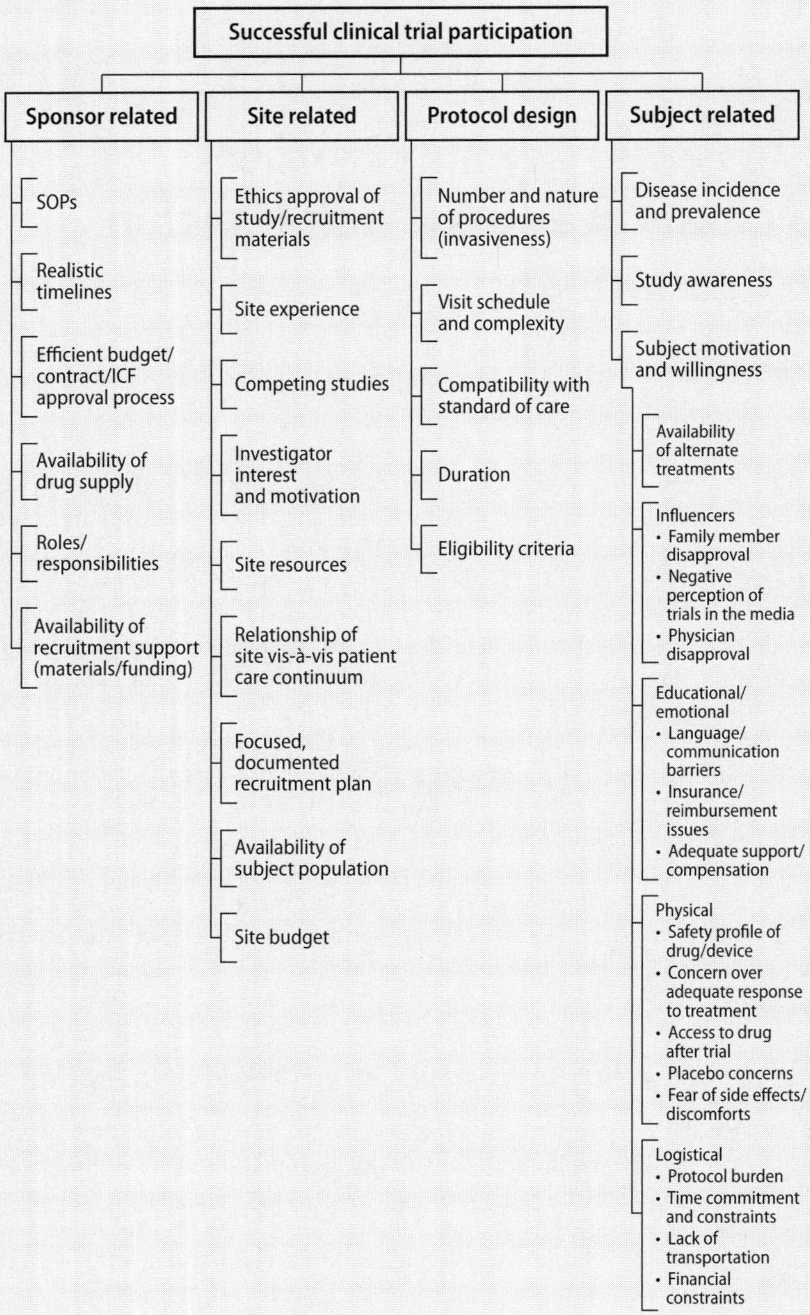

Source: Clinical Performance Partners Inc., 2007

interests and motivations. Combine this with the fact that subjects come from diverse geographic regions, socioeconomic statuses and cultural backgrounds. Further adding to the difficulties is the necessity to involve multiple investigative sites, also from different regions with different standards of care, resources, infrastructures and approaches to patient recruitment, retention and study conduct.

A Complex Problem Becomes Even More Daunting

As if these challenges were not enough, protocols themselves are becoming more complex and burdensome. Data from the Tufts Center for the Study of Drug Development indicates the number of procedures, eligibility criteria, case report form pages and amendments are all increasing[1]. This not only adds to the work burden at the sites, but also, the more complex a protocol, the more difficult it is to enroll and retain subjects.

The Tufts CSDD report further suggests that the financial burden associated with resolving each amendment is approximately $450,000 not to mention a 61-day cycle time. It concludes that nearly half of all amendments occur *before* the first patient dose and that 40% of all amendments are considered completely unavoidable.

Given all these challenges and complexities, one can quickly see that ensuring a "good fit" among the protocol, multiple sites and subjects can be daunting. That's where the protocol evaluation and site feasibility assessment processes come in. Gaining an appreciation for which aspects of the study design will drive enrollment success at the study and site level early in the protocol development process is key to avoiding amendments and "rescue mode" once the study has been launched.

Figure 2: Rising protocol complexity, burden and impact (all TAs, all phases)

	2000-03	2004-07	Percentage change
Unique procedures per protocol (median)	20.5	28.2	38%
Total procedures per protocol (median)	105.9	158.1	49%
Total investigative site work burden (median units)	28.9	44.6	54%
Total eligibility criteria	31	49	58%

Source: Tufts CSDD, <csdd.tufts.edu>

Figure 3: Impact of protocol complexity and burden (all TAs, all phases)

	Less complex protocols	More complex protocols	Difference
Number of case report form pages per protocol (median)	55	180	+38%
Study volunteer enrollment rates	75%	59%	-21%
Study volunteer retention rates	69%	48%	-30%
Time from protocol ready to last patient last visit (LPLV)	413 weeks	714 weeks	+72%
Number of amendments	1.9	3.2	+68%

Source: Tufts CSDD, <csdd.tufts.edu>

The "Typical" Protocol Evaluation and Feasibility Process

Ensuring a good fit among sites, protocol and patient population requires careful assessment of many factors. Typically, biopharmaceutical companies (sponsors) and contract research organizations (CROs) have followed a process that concurrently evaluates country and site feasibility while the protocol concept is being finalized. Scientific advisory boards and input from Key Opinion Leaders (KOLs) are used to validate the scientific soundness of the study and ensure the medical feasibility of the protocol. At the country level, country managers and local experts evaluate any potential conflicts with the study design and standard of care in the region, or issues associated with access to comparator drugs, to determine if the study is viable to conduct in the country. Interested and appropriate countries then have the opportunity to participate in the site feasibility process, which focuses on identifying suitable investigators to be considered for site selection.

The site feasibility assessment process routinely involves the distribution of feasibility or pre-trial questionnaires in paper or electronic format. Site representatives (typically research coordinators, site directors or business development personnel) complete the questionnaires and the sponsor/CRO evaluates the responses. This drives the "short listing" process, from which potential investigators under a more robust site qualification process (including on-site, pre-study visits) confirm site qualifications. From there, the final site list is determined around the time the protocol is finalized and the site initiation process ensues.

A detailed review of the parameters and steps associated with site feasibility and selection are beyond the scope of this discussion. From a patient recruitment perspective, however, feasibility questionnaires generally ask a few questions related to the volume of patients seen within the site's clinic or practice, the number of competing trials and the estimated number of

Figure 4: A simplistic representation of the "typical" process

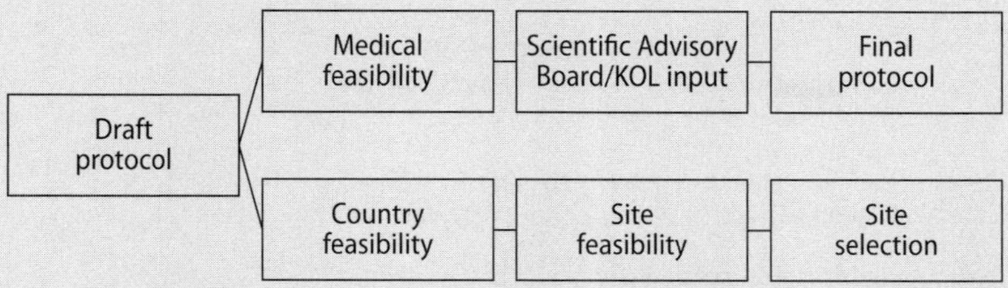

Source: Clinical Performance Partners, Inc.

patients the site believes can be recruited in the planned enrollment period. Figure 5 provides a representation of the typical patient enrollment questions included in the feasibility questionnaire.

This questionnaire represents the type of questions in a "typical" enrollment feasibility survey. Sometimes the questions may be vague or open to interpretation, and in other cases the grammar itself may be confusing. In many cases the actual questions either lead to sites over-estimating their enrollment, or the questions don't actually help the sponsor convert the answers into any meaningful forecasts. For example, just knowing that the site has a computerized patient database ("yes or no") does little, if anything, to help the sponsor understand how the database might be leveraged to analyze the inclusion /exclusion criteria or to accelerate recruitment.

Sites, on the other hand, vary in their approaches to the feasibility assessment process. Some have robust internal review processes in which representatives from various functional roles (investigators, coordinators, research pharmacists, lab technicians, ethics committee members) vet the protocol to identify the interest and feasibility of conducting the trial at their institution. Other sites may take a cursory look at the protocol synopsis, inquire about the investigator's interest and complete the questionnaire without delving into the eligibility criteria and operational factors and burdens that can affect successful study implementation. Regardless of the approach, the bottom line is that sites are asked to estimate the number of subjects who would likely qualify within the planned enrollment period.

Sponsors may compare and contrast the site's estimates to historical enrollment performance but, at the end of the day, most sponsors and CROs discount enrollment estimates by 25%, 33% or 50% to "hedge their bets" against potential over inflation by investigators eager to be selected to participate in the trial.

Figure 5: Common patient recruitment-related questions in a feasibility questionnaire

Patient enrollment	
Please provide an estimate of how many subjects with the stated indication do you see at your institution every month:	
Please provide an estimate of how many subjects with the stated indication will you be able to enroll over a year:	
Please provide an estimate of how many subjects potentially meet the inclusion/exclusion criteria for this study:	
Do you have a computerized patient database?	❍ Yes ❍ No

For your past 3 studies, please describe:

	Indication	Enrollment goal	Actual number screened	Actual number randomized	Actual number completed
1					
2					
3					

Are you currently conducting or planning to conduct, in the next 6 months, a competing study for the same indication?	❍ Yes ❍ No
How will patients be allocated if they meet eligibility criteria for more than one study?	

Submit Cancel

Source: www.vistasurveys.com

The "Typical" Result

Sadly, the typical result of this process, from a site enrollment standpoint, is that less than 10% of sites deliver what they estimate in the feasibility questionnaire according to data[2], regardless of study phase or therapeutic area.

Despite years of failure, the biopharmaceutical industry has continued to follow this traditional process, which has resulted in poor site enrollment performance, chronic delays in achieving on-time enrollment and a growing number of amendments and other interventions applied to "rescue and rejuvenate" studies that fall behind.

Figure 6: Typical site recruitment pattern

Percentage of sites	Number or percentage of evaluable patients enrolled
15-20% of sites	Enroll 0 patients
30% of sites	Enroll 5% of evaluable patients
20% of sites	Enroll 25% of evaluable patients
30% of sites	Enroll 70% of evaluable patients

Source: McKinsey & Co., 2004; Tufts CSDD, <csdd.tufts.edu>, 2007

A Flawed Process in Need of Fixing

To uncover opportunities to improve the process, we must first evaluate where the process fails. Some key root cause issues for which the process fails in terms of generating highly predictive enrollment forecasts include, but are not limited to, the following:

- The site feasibility assessment process is focused on selecting sites, not identifying challenges and opportunities related to optimizing patient recruitment and retention.
- The feasibility questionnaires don't ask questions that drive enrollment and execution success and often are focused on other aspects related to site qualifications.
- Various and multiple stakeholders at the site (investigators, coordinators, pharmacists, etc.) are rarely involved in the feasibility assessment process.
- Many sites don't systematically evaluate the protocol and rely on sponsor/CRO questionnaires to drive their review and analysis of the protocol.
- Feasibility assessment is subjective in nature and not objective or "evidence based."
- Enrollment validation activities are not performed to confirm enrollment potential.
- Feasibility assessments are based on the protocol synopsis or draft protocol and not revisited when the final protocol and budget are available.
- Not enough information is provided to sites at the time of the assessment.
- Sites are not provided enough time to complete a thorough analysis.
- Sites are not asked to provide or given an opportunity to provide input on operational aspects of the study or other barriers affecting recruitment and study execution success.

- There is too much dependency on tools (questionnaires vs. checklists) vs. conversations to discuss recruitment and execution issues and recommendations.

Ensuring a Good Fit—What Will it Take?

How do we go about ensuring a good fit among the protocol, sites and patient population? What will it take to be successful and where should we focus our efforts in the protocol evaluation and feasibility assessment process? To begin, we need a clear understanding of what we are trying to accomplish with the evaluation and feasibility process and a clear definition of the terms protocol evaluation and feasibility.

The American Heritage® Dictionary defines feasible as: "capable of being accomplished or brought about; possible: *a feasible plan.*" Synonyms for feasible include achievable, attainable, doable, possible, practicable, realizable, viable or workable.

In terms of protocol evaluation, there are many factors to evaluate that determine whether a given protocol is capable of being executed on time and on budget. A systematic and structured evaluation of the scientific and medical feasibility; ethical feasibility; operational, technical, financial and contractual feasibility; and recruitment and retention feasibility are all required at both the country and site levels. The protocol evaluation should comprise an assessment of key "red flag" issues that can affect enrollment and study execution success, along with recommendations to overcome these issues. Finally, a determination should be made regarding the potential impact the changes would have on timely and predictable execution. An "executability scorecard" such as that depicted in Figure 7 provides an "at-a-glance" visual representation of the key at-risk areas and rates the likelihood of successful execution based on the protocol as written, with changes and the final score based on incorporation of any protocol modifications.

In terms of the feasibility analysis, the improved process should:

- Provide ample information and adequate time to conduct a proper analysis.
- Clearly differentiate an evaluation of whether the study is "doable" from an assessment of site interest and capabilities (both of which are important to the site selection process but may not relate to an assessment of protocol feasibility).
- Be performed early in the protocol development stage and independent of the site selection process to avoid a situation in which sites tell the sponsor what they think the sponsor wants to hear to be selected to participate in the trial.
- Involve a dialogue and discussion with all relevant stakeholders about enrollment risks and opportunities.

Figure 7: Protocol executability scorecard

Executability score	Protocol as written	With suggested revisions	Final score based on accepted changes
Study participation interest/Motivation	!	✓	✓
Scientific interest	✓	✓	✓
Scientific/Medical feasibility	!	✓	✓
Risk: Benefit, ethical, safety, feasibilty	✓	✓	✓
Patient availability	!	!	!
Recruitment feasibility: Site perspective	!	✓	!
Recruitment feasibility: Patient perspective	!	✓	✓
Compliance/retention	✓	✓	✓
Operational/infrastructure feasibility	!	✓	✓
Operational/technical feasibility	✓	✓	✓
Financial feasibility	×	✓	!
Contractual feasibility	×	✓	!
Total score (Percent of maximum)	**74%**	**89%**	**83%**
Confidence level that protocol can be successfully implemented within specified timeline	**Moderate**	**High**	**Moderately high**

Key	Not feasible	At risk	Feasible
	×	!	✓

Source: Centerphase Solutions, 2010

- Incorporate feedback from a representative sample of different types of sites and subject matter experts around the globe and ideally incorporate input and feedback from potential patients (i.e., market research and patient focus groups).

Figure 8: Key questions site personnel should evaluate during the patient recruitment feasibility assessment process

Patient availability	For patients in our existing population (pool) who meet the diagnostic and eligibility criteria required in the protocol, how many of these patients are NOT currently participating in other studies?
	How many of these patients are likely to be able to attend all protocol required visits (e.g., they are within a reasonable geographic region to be able to participate)?
	Are we aware of any other clinical research studies taking place in our institution or city that may complete for patients in this study?
	Will the protocol require a treatment-naïve population? If so, how will this affect the availability of the patients as well as the recruitment plan and budget?
	How easy or difficult will it be to find subjects for this study?
Patient accessibility	How easy or difficult will it be to enroll subjects for this study? How many and which sources will be needed?
	When is enrollment expected to begin?
	What is the duration of the enrollment period?
	Can the investigator enroll more than the allocated number of subjects? If so, under what criteria (e.g., competitive enrollment, after certain block size of subjects has been enrolled, etc.)?
	What are the expected pre-screen and screen-fail/loss ratios? How does this compare to our recent experience and our estimates?
	What other recruitment or referral sources will we require to identify and obtain patients for this study?
	Will we need to interface with other professionals in the institution or community to identify potential candidates? What is "in it for them" to identify subjects for this study? Will we need to compensate these professionals for their time and effort? If so, are there any institutional policies on the nature and amount of compensation allowed?
	Based on past experience what have been the most effective recruitment strategies?
	What was the cost of these strategies in past studies?
	What type of recruitment and/or retention support (if any) will be provided by the sponsor/CRO (e.g., centralized advertising, telephone screening service, internet advertising)?
	Does the institution or IRB/ERC restrict or limit subject payment/compensation? If so, what are the limits? Will this affect our ability to enroll the required number of subjects in the required timeframe?
	To what extent will the sponsor/CRO pay for subjects who are screened but don't qualify?
	Are vulnerable populations involved (children, prisoners, educationally challenged) that may require additional IRB and recruitment protections?

Figure 8: Key questions site personnel should evaluate during the patient recruitment feasibility assessment process

Patient alacrity	What percent of accessible patients are likely to be interested in participating?
	What do we think it will take to make the study attractive to potential subjects (e.g., recruitment or retention "incentives," compensation, recognition items, etc.)?
	How "burdensome" is this study from the subjects' perspective? What is the duration of the study? How many visits will subjects need to make to the site? Will this study require subjects to miss work or school?
	What are the nature and number of procedures subjects must undergo? How many are invasive?
	What things could we recommend to the sponsor to make the study less burdensome for patients?
	What is the expected consent/refusal ratio? How does this compare to our recent experience in similar studies and to our estimates?
	What is the expected dropout ratio? How does this compare to our estimates?
	How do we plan to keep subjects interested in participating? Are we planning to use any retention incentives? Will the sponsor/CRO provide financial support for these? What is the likelihood that the IRB/IEC will approve such incentives?
	How do we plan to ensure subjects keep their visits (e.g., send reminder postcards, have staff call subjects the day prior to their visit)? What implications will these activities have for staff time and the budget (e.g., will the sponsor/CRO fund these activities)?
	How do we plan to monitor subject compliance with protocol-required activities and the dosing regimen?

Source: Clinical Performance Partners, Inc.

- Leverage Operational Advisory Boards (OABs), protocol simulation and optimization workshops provide the ideal forum to gather input from a variety of subject matter experts in a structured and organized fashion.
- Be designed to uncover the key characteristics that will define a high-performing site for the specific trial that can be used to inform the ultimate site selection strategy.
- Incorporate protocol simulation and optimization activities to "de-risk" the protocol from an operational and executability standpoint.
- Focus on the three "As" of recruitment success: patient **availability**, patient **accessibility** and patient **alacrity**.

Beyond asking one or two questions about the volume of patients seen in the site's practice in a given time period and the number of competing trials, sites should perform a much more robust assessment of the factors affecting enrollment success including, but not limited to, the key questions outlined in Figure 8.

While there are many opportunities to overhaul the protocol evaluation, feasibility and site selection process, the remainder of this chapter will focus specifically on ways to enhance the accuracy and predictability of enrollment forecasting and performance.

Assessing and Confirming Patient Availability

The first step in an improved process is to confirm that patients who meet the strict (and growing number of) eligibility criteria actually exist within a given region or site. Whereas the traditional process of estimating enrollment is based on "guesstimates" by the sites combined with an evaluation of historical performance and the competitive landscape, the new and improved process is much more evidence based.

Disease prevalence and incidence rates are a good starting point from which to determine the general percentage of the population in a given country or community that might have the condition of interest. Heat maps provide a nice way to visualize the population density in certain regions and can prove useful for targeting site selection activities.

An assessment of historical enrollment performance can provide additional clues to the estimated enrollment potential for a given site and/or region. These high-level estimates need to be quantified at the individual site level or, at a minimum, for the various site types participating in the trial.

A recruitment funnel or "leaky pipe" analysis is performed to determine the loss ratios and reasons across various stages of the recruitment funnel (pre-screening, consent refusals, screen failures and post-randomization dropouts). This can be performed at the site level using a manual review process of a sample of charts or through a more sophisticated analysis of de-identified information from various electronic medical record (EMR) systems, Health Information Exchanges (HIEs) and other data warehouses at both the site and regional levels. These technologies offer the promise and potential of combining data across multiple sites and regions to characterize the conversion ratios from available patients to enrolled patients at the site, country and study levels.

To encourage compliance with good clinical practice guidelines[3], it is becoming more routine for sponsors to request evidence from sites of the available patient population within their clinics and communities. Several articles have described the recruitment funnel analysis and enrollment forecasting methods as a means of performing more data-driven approaches to estimating availability of patients within a given region and validating enrollment potential at a given site[4, 5]. Individual site estimates, now validated through an evidence-based approach, are rolled up to create a study-wide forecast. This combined "top down" and "bottom up" approach enables study teams to develop more realistic and accurate enrollment projections.

Figure 9: Representative recruitment funnel showing a cohort of patients residing within 50 miles of Mayo Clinic

Recruitment funnel ("reasonable" estimate)

12-month enrollment period

Patient funnel: 50 miles of Mayo Clinic

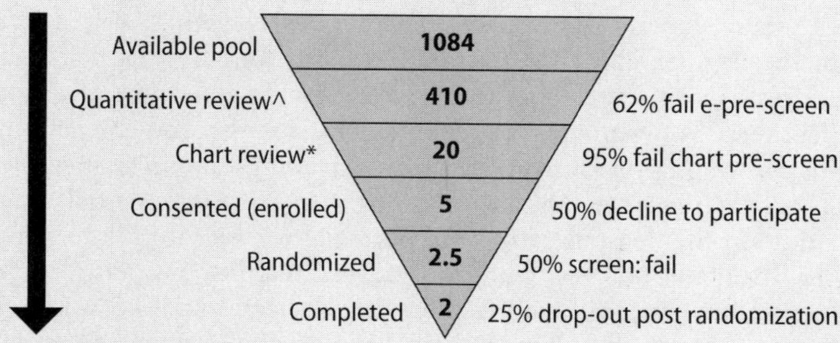

Primary loss reasons:

Pre-screening (database)

- Currently on medication A or B (-38%)
- History of disease W (-18%)
- History of disease X (-1%)
- Exclusionary criteria Y (-10%)
- Exclusionary criteria Z (-6%)
- No research authorization (-11%)

Pre-screening (e-chart)

- Unstable medical condition (-55%)
- Criteria J did not meet required criteria scores (-40%)
- Patient on meds that would require washout (-40%)
- Diagnosis of study disease could not be confirmed (-20%)

Consent

- Study burdens (burden 1, burden 2, burden 3)
- Unwillingness to wash-out of medications
- Competing trial opportunity
- Additional medication burden
- General reluctance to participate in clinical trial; demand on caregiver

Screening

- Baseline criteria K scores
- Lab/EKG findings
- Non-compliance with diary

Notes:

^Identify Conversion Ratio=75:1: Identify ~75 patients with study disease to randomize 1

*Approach Conversion Ratio=4:1: Approach ~4 patients with study disease to randomize 1

Database pre-screening loss ratios represent successive (i.e., sequential) losses from the prior criteria

Chart review loss ratios represent overall loss ratios

Source: Clinical Performance Partners, Inc.

Figure 9 shows the results of a recruitment funnel analysis performed at Mayo Clinic in 2010. Figure 9 shows the "reverse funnel" calculations and impact to overall study enrollment based on the assumptions and loss ratios applied from the Mayo Clinic population.

Further, this data mining process allows the study team to "pressure test" the protocol and determine which inclusion and exclusion criteria are driving the biggest loss ratios along the recruitment funnel. Discussions with subject matter experts regarding the viability of changing certain criteria (i.e., medically justifiable changes) and the ability to run "what if" scenarios and perform sensitivity analyses help to ascertain the impact of changing certain criteria. For example, does expanding the range around a certain lab value or allowing a previously restrictive medication result in an incremental (e.g., 1-2% difference) or substantial (15-20%) increase in potential patients?

In addition to "demonstrating the potential for recruiting the required number of suitable subjects within the agreed recruitment period," the recruitment funnel analysis enables sites and sponsors to answer a key question: Can a sufficient number of eligible subjects be recruited from within the investigators' own practices? If not, the gap between the potential number of subjects available at the site and the ideal target enrollment can be determined. This will influence decisions about whether additional sites (and possibly countries) should be identified to fulfill the gap or whether a recruitment support program should be developed (at the site and/or study level) to bring in patients from external sources.

Evaluating Patient Accessibility and Enrollability

Beyond knowing if patients exist who meet the eligibility criteria, it's important to determine how accessible the patient population is and how enrollable the study is. Patient accessibility is determined through a systematic exploration of all of the various sources of patients. Generally speaking, there are three primary sources of patients: those who exist within an investigator's own clinic or institution, patients who can be accessed through other healthcare professionals and those who reside in the community-at-large.

"Patient Pathways" or flow diagrams are helpful tools for understanding how patients navigate the healthcare system in a given country or community. They enable sites and sponsors to understand the access points (i.e., where the patient enters the healthcare system), which healthcare practitioners they may encounter, who may be a potential source of patients and/or where opportunities exist to educate prospective subjects about clinical research and the study in general.

Assuming not all patients will come from within the investigator's own pool of patients, it's important to determine:

- Where they will come from
- What will be done to identify and attract patients into the study

Figure 10: Reverse funnel analysis showing the number of patients needed at a given site (and extrapolated to the overall study) who will be required to complete the enrollment period

Anticipated recruitment funnel required to randomize 8 patients/site
("Reverse funnel analysis" applying Centerphase-Mayo ratios)

Assumptions:

- 12-month enrollment period
- "Reasonable" loss ratios
- Reasonable geographic distance of patients from site

Patient funnel: 50 miles from site

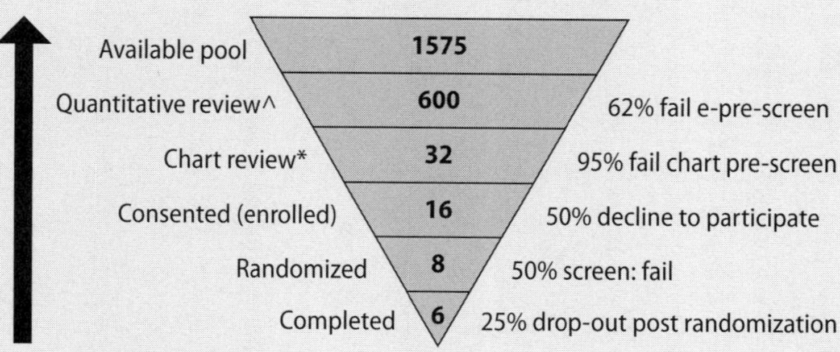

Applying Centerphase estimates, a given will need access to ~1,575 patients to successfully randomize 8 subjects per year. This translates to access to some 35,438 patients to enroll the required 180 subjects in the study.

Source: Clinical Performance Partners, Inc.

- How the potential participants will learn about the study opportunity
- What tools and methods will be used to raise awareness of the study

Assessing enrollability of the trial involves a careful analysis of the factors that make enrollment challenging so that appropriate mitigation plans can be developed. For example, if the challenge is finding patients, then outreach and awareness programs may be needed. Challenges related to study burdens and inconveniences might require patient retention programs (assuming the protocol visit schedule and procedures cannot be modified). Issues related to study design, placebo or safety concerns might be mitigated with supplemental patient education materials and/or development and rehearsal of important messages.

The use of operational advisory boards, simulation panels and structured interview techniques (e.g., Baysean interview/probability encoding) enable sponsors to determine the best and worst case enrollment scenarios[5,6]. Conducting a thorough root-cause analysis of the factors driving recruitment up or down is a critical and often missed step in the recruitment planning process.

Figure 11: Illustrative patient pathway—rheumatoid arthritis example

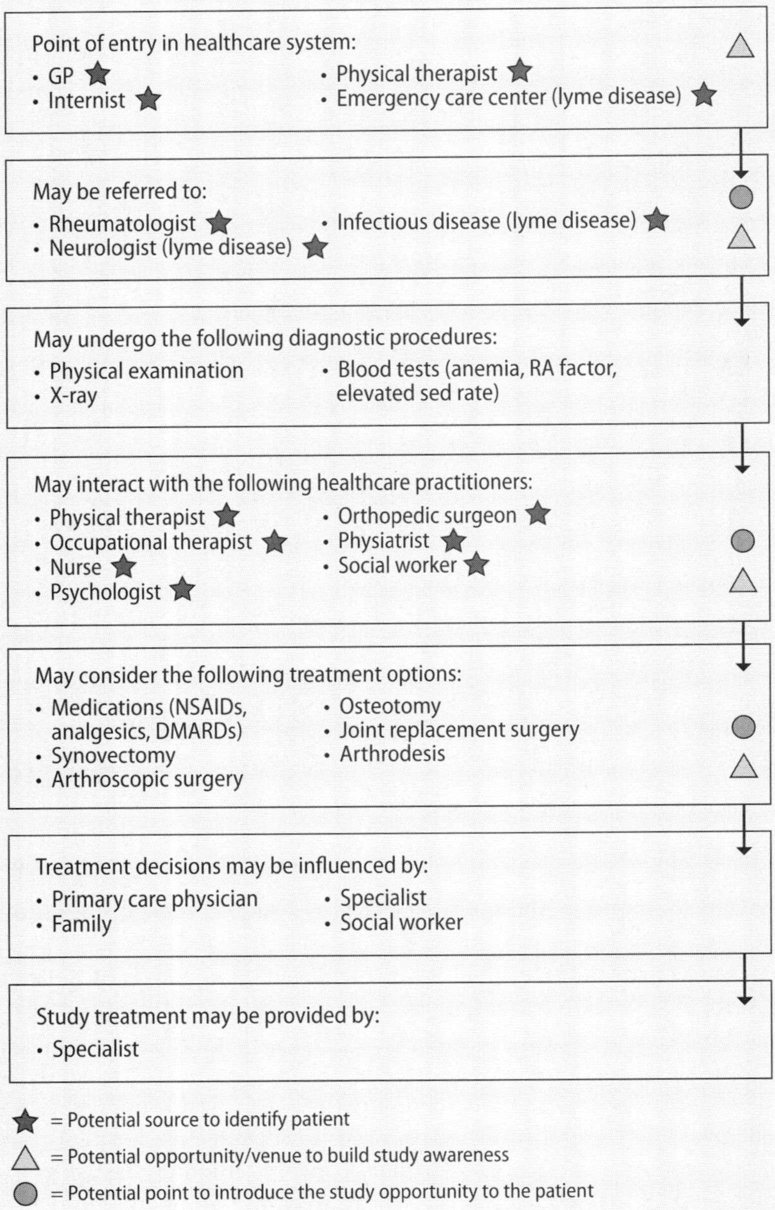

Source: Clinical Performance Partners, Inc.

Answering such questions will enable the sponsors and sites to determine the ease or difficulty of enrolling the study, what strategies and tactics will be needed to support the awareness and outreach efforts and ultimately support the development of a proactive recruitment and retention plan. Without this, sponsors are often tempted to develop study awareness and recruitment campaigns designed to "fill the funnel" of patients, whereas the "real" recruitment problem may revolve around "managing the leaks" of patients through the pre-screening, consent, screening and post-randomization processes.

Understanding Patient Alacrity

The most challenging aspect of the protocol evaluation and site-level feasibility assessment process as it pertains to recruitment planning and forecasting is assessing patient eagerness, willingness and motivation to participate in a trial.

The quantitative evaluations described above should be coupled with qualitative discussions with subject matter experts (along with benchmarking of similar and recent trial experience) to assess the consent refusal and dropout ratios, which highlight the impact of protocol burdens on patient and caregiver willingness to participate in a trial.

Even more important than tapping into site perspectives and historical information, sponsors should conduct market research and patient focus groups to gain a better understanding of patient needs, motivations, interests, fears and concerns as they pertain to study participation. Patient recruitment service providers offer the ability to conduct different types of market research. If time and resources prohibit an in-depth, study-specific focus group, at a minimum sponsors and sites should review the published literature to gain insights on the general issues affecting patient willingness to participate.

For example, sponsors may estimate that only 20% of the pre-qualified patients who are approached about the study will decline the opportunity to participate (i.e., consent-refusal ratio of 20% or consent/ conversion ratio of 80%). Market research, however, might suggest that based on the study burdens, risk-benefit ratio, competing trials, availability of alternative treatments and the like, closer to 75% of patients might decline. The impact of underestimating the consent-refusal ratio can have a significant bearing on enrollment forecasts and timelines.

Conclusion

Patient recruitment and retention in clinical trials are complex processes. Success is driven by a realistic or feasible protocol (the more patient and site-friendly the better), interested, qualified and capable sites that have access to the appropriate patient population and a well thought-out and proactive recruitment and retention plan. Investing in a robust protocol analysis and feasibility assessment process to address the three "As" of successful enrollment (patient availability, accessibility and alacrity) are essential elements to set a study up for success. In this chapter we have outlined opportunities

Figure 12: Comparative analysis

Shows the impact of the consent-refusal ratio on the total volume of patients required to randomize 10 patients at a site over a nine-month enrollment period

Reverse or "bottom up" funnel calculations

	20% Consent refusal ratio	75% Consent refusal ratio
Funnel parameters and stages	**Values**	
Enrollment period (months)	9	9
Number of sites	1	1
Number of patients that will need to be identified	**53**	**171**
Percent lost during pre-screening	.33	.33
Percent declined to participate	.2	.75
Percent lost during screening	.65	.65
Percent drop-out post randomization	.25	.25
Funnel calculations	**Projected values**	
Patients that need to be identified	53	171
Pre-screen qualified	36	114
Consented (enrolled)	29	29
Randomized	10	10
Completed	8	8
Number enrolled/month	3	3

	20% Consent refusal ratio	75% Consent refusal ratio	20% Consent refusal ratio	75% Consent refusal ratio
Per-site estimates (approximate)	**Overall targets**		**Monthly estimates**	
Number needed to be identified	53.3	170.6	5.9	19.0
Number needed to be pre-screened	35.7	114.3	4.0	12.7
Number needed to be consented	28.6	28.6	3.2	3.2
Number needed to be randomized	10.0	10.0	1.1	1.1

Source: Clinical Performance Partners, Inc.

to transform the traditional feasibility assessment process from flawed and failed to data-driven and predictive. While protocol design and patient recruitment planning will always require a blend of "art and science," EMR-enabled technologies and more structured quantitative analyses combined with qualitative input from sites and patients provide the necessary ingredients for ensuring an optimized protocol is developed—one that can successfully be enrolled on time and with minimal deviations or amendments.

Author Biography

Beth Harper is president of Clinical Performance Partners, a clinical research consulting firm specializing in enrollment and site performance management. Previously she was Chief Clinical Officer of Centerphase Solutions, a technology-enabled consultancy specializing in protocol optimization services, and Senior Vice President at D. Anderson and Company, a patient recruitment and retention firm. Beth has also worked at Merck Research Labs and MedTrials, a Dallas-based CRO. In addition to her 28 years of clinical research experience, she is an Adjunct Assistant Professor at George Washington University and has published and presented extensively in the areas of study feasibility, site selection, patient recruitment and protocol optimization. Beth is currently a member of ACRP's Editorial Advisory Board. She received her B.S. in Occupational Therapy from the University of Wisconsin and an MBA from the University of Texas.

References

1. Getz et al. Assessing the Impact of Protocol Design Change on Clinical Trial Performance. American Journal of Therapeutics. 2008 15 (5); 450-457.

2. Reuter, S. How Effective Are Research Site Questionnaires in Predicting Site Performance? George Washington University - Masters Degree Thesis - 2005

3. ICH GCP Section 4.2.1 stipulates that "The investigator should be able to demonstrate (e.g., based on retrospective data) a potential for recruiting the required number of suitable subjects within the agreed recruitment period."

4. Harper, B. Projecting Realistic Enrollment Rates: Principles and Methodology. The Monitor. 2004 – Winter Issue. 15 – 18.

5. Harper, B. and D. Zuckerman. No Virginia, There is No Enrollment Problem: Bursting the Myth of Late Enrollment. The Monitor. 2008 – October. 33-38.

6. Harper, B. Gathering and Implementing Feasibility Data into Protocol Design: Lessons Learned and Realistic Outcomes. Presentation at Barnett Clinical Summit – October 2011.

CHAPTER FOUR

Metrics Reporting and Objective Measurement of Recruitment Outcomes

By John Benbrook

The Evolution of Outcome Measurements

Since the introduction of formalized patient recruitment efforts for clinical trials, study teams have increasingly pressed for outcomes measurements. Although stakeholders have long agreed we must find a way to measure performance to determine ROI and advance recruitment methodologies, the necessary data collection mechanisms and supporting behaviors have been conspicuously absent. However, innovations in technology and intense economic pressures have propelled us into a new era. We can now generate meaningful patient recruitment metrics and accumulate broad performance benchmarks for a variety of recruitment interventions.

It has not been a minor evolution. In the early years of recruitment outreach, many programs were heavily based in traditional media advertising, with placements made by sites and recruitment groups according to their preferences and how they defined success. Such placements were rarely consistent from site to site or group to group. Looking back, we see that traditional media's limited ability to tightly target outreach, coupled with the dispersed management of programs, served to dilute the effectiveness of recruitment tactics and delay the development of recruitment metrics. In addition, the lack of recruitment benchmarks today, in part, stems from the surprising number of study teams that for a number of years considered recruitment outcomes to be competitive intelligence—so much so that they would withhold results from the group managing the recruitment program for the study.

Recruitment funds also were often allocated as a line item in each site's study budget, with no distinction made between funds to support the placement of direct-to-patient advertising versus assistance with internal chart review. Sites also were not aggressively required to report ROI. Although it seems unthinkable to us now that sites would receive funds for placing advertising and not be required to report response activity and conversion rates, it is important to remember that in fairly recent history, expectations, dynamics and pressures were markedly different.

For instance, study teams were understandably quite sensitive to the additional effort required by site staff to adopt electronic case report forms and other electronic trial management systems. In that environment, it was a challenge to garner support for asking site staff to perform extra tasks. Making recruitment funds available could help maintain or even improve a site's commitment to the study, but attaching formal outcomes reporting requirements would likely dampen that effect. In the case of local advertising, sites may have kept an approximate count of calls received, but inquiries about the source of enrolled patients consistently yielded reports that the lion's share of participants were identified from the sites' databases. Despite seemingly poor performance, many sites continued to eagerly request advertising funds. This disconnect, coupled with the spectacular failures of some large, perhaps misguided media buys, created an environment in which study teams and recruitment strategists struggled to secure approval for outreach that they believed would produce results but could not support with data.

In the early 2000s, Internet-based patient recruitment tactics began to take off and, shortly thereafter, Internet promotion analytics gave us more precise referral source tracking and greater trending capabilities. With the rise of these analytics, as well as an unprecedented volume of response activity data, suddenly we had a new, broad-reaching medium for attracting patients to studies and raising awareness among the healthcare and advocacy communities that was consistently measurable. We had data! Patient recruitment conferences dedicated breakout sessions to understanding terms such as page views, click-throughs and bounce rates. Finally, patient recruitment began moving into the comfort zone of those with budget approval authority—a place with data points, pie charts and histograms.

Simultaneous to the Internet explosion, an escalation in strategic sourcing began driving discussions of performance-based contracts for patient recruitment, whereby recruitment-support providers are compensated based on the number of patients referred to or enrolled in a study. While this raises several interesting questions about the accountability for a trial's enrollment performance, because pay-for-performance pricing requires metrics, it has fueled willingness on the part of study teams to make enrollment activity data and outcomes available to those executing recruitment programs.

Outcomes Measurement Planning

Now, more than a full decade into the new century, the good news/bad news is that the remaining obstacles to achieving robust recruitment metrics are based primarily in behaviors. On the sponsor side, this includes study teams' willingness to integrate a recruitment metrics plan into study setup. Like so much of clinical trial management, recruitment metrics is 80 percent planning and 20 percent execution. It takes time to think through not just what *can* be measured, but what *should* be measured—and then *how* it should be measured, *when* it should be measured and *who* should measure it. It takes time and advance planning to set up the data exchange, collection systems and processes. Although there are signs that recruitment planning is steadily becoming part of clinical trial management best practice, it is not yet the standard. It is critical that metrics planning be supported with clear, consistent communication of a firm expectation for all stakeholders, especially study sites, to make the collection of the required data a priority and to report the required information fully and without delay.

The success of most recruitment metrics plans is dependent to some degree on the active participation of study sites; specifically, their willingness to report outcomes and the diligence with which they report them. Unfortunately, this historically has been a more complex dynamic than it needs to be. Some sites view the implementation of a recruitment program as an implied criticism of their ability to satisfy the performance expectations of the study, and they may feel threatened or perturbed by requests to provide detailed reports of screening and recruitment activities. This can also occur among CRO teams, which significantly compounds the challenge of securing the data needed for metrics. Ironically, correlating increases in enrollment to indirect, non-outreach tactics—such as coaching site staff on speaking points for consenting patients and assisting with chart reviews—is less dependent on sites reporting recruitment activity data than the concrete, direct-to-patient outreach tactics that drive referrals to sites. Of course, study teams are usually more successful in obtaining approval for the direct outreach tactics, because the results feel more tangible. Nevertheless, success often comes down to what happens at the site. This is why recruitment programs in which sites interface directly with those implementing recruitment tactics on their behalf consistently achieve stronger metrics and outcomes.

The most significant challenges to establishing and executing a metrics plan often include:

- **Time Constraints and Cost Pressures.** Limited resources not only narrow the field of available recruitment tactics but also often restrict the ability to collect and analyze performance data. Ideally, a metrics plan allows for pre/post-intervention or cohort group comparative analyses. As cost or time constraints force an analysis further away from direct comparisons, the analysis loses strength and validity.

- **Study Variances.** As tempting as it is to base recruitment performance predictions and recruitment strategy selection on experience with past trials, we must keep in mind that no two trials are sufficiently the same to guarantee outcomes—adjustments need to be made even for the same trial repeated a short time later, because the landscape is different at each point in time. Therefore, every recruitment program has its own unique mix of strategies and tactics, and the metrics plan needs to be customized accordingly. This necessary variance is a primary challenge to the industry's ability to identify trends and formulate generalizations that will hold across indications, study types, patient populations, geography and time. Having a mix of central and decentralized response pathways (i.e., the call to action for Internet promotion is to visit a study web site, and the call to action for community outreach is to contact the study site directly) creates an uneven metrics field, with one having much richer, more consistent data than the other, and limits the comparative analyses that can be performed.

- **Geographic Locations.** Metrics plans for multinational studies often need to account for two common variances encountered with global recruitment programs: 1) differences in the recruitment tactics implemented across countries, preventing "apples to apples" performance comparisons, and 2) legal restrictions on the collection of data from patients who respond to outreach. It is important to note that confusion about which data can and cannot be collected by each country has created a misalignment between actual data protection requirements and self-imposed restrictions based on conservative preferences of the study sponsor's legal and/or regulatory team. For instance, although it is not as easy to store patient data in France and Spain because of their data protection laws, most countries do not prohibit other forms of data collection. Too often, this results in missed opportunities to collect valuable metrics.
- **Data Types and Definitions.** Even when there is uniformity in the tactics implemented among trials, countries and sites, inconsistencies regarding which data are captured, the detail with which they are collected and the respective completeness of the data sets can all result in censored analyses. Date formats should be standardized and exact definitions for key events, such as site activation, screening and enrollment date, all need to be established.
- **Tactic Measurability.** Not all tactics are equally measureable. Of note, some "soft" tactics that historically have been excluded from metrics plans, such patient education materials and informed consent aids, are now showing strong correlation to screening and recruitment activity.

The development of a recruitment metrics plan can be divided into seven steps.

1. Ensure Up-Front Commitment From All Stakeholders.

The metrics plan needs to be developed before recruitment begins and have the support of all those who will contribute at each step. This will help prevent changes in the metrics plan or disagreement about the validity of the metrics results at analysis. If data collection for a metrics plan is started after recruitment has begun, the pre-program data needed for a valid analysis may

Figure 1: The seven steps of a recruitment metrics plan

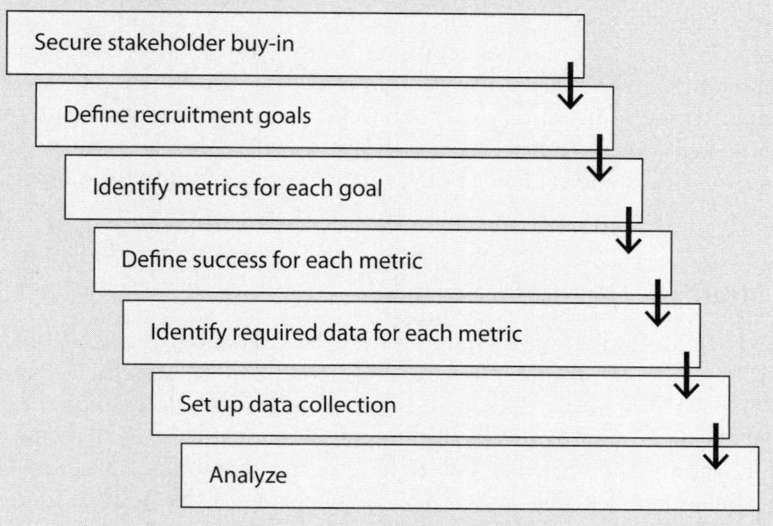

Source: MMG

not be available. If there is disagreement on the value of the metrics and a lack of understanding regarding the critical pathway to securing them, the risk of missing data increases.

2. Define Recruitment Goals.

The overall goal of the recruitment program and the goals of individual tactics need to be defined and prioritized. Some tactics may be designed to build awareness within a physician community for a global, multi-protocol program. The purpose of other tactics may be to aid study sites in communicating with patients about the study. A tactic may be effective in building a referral network or increasing screenings at study sites. At the program level, the goal may be to accelerate enrollment or to meet enrollment targets.

Once the list of program and tactic goals is created, it should be prioritized by importance to the metrics analysis. Time and resource investment levels in metrics-related activities can be determined based on the importance of the goal compared to other study/tactic goals and the availability of measurable outcomes for that goal (discussed below). For example, investing in measuring the outcome of a large media campaign should significantly outweigh investing in measuring the impact of a single study brochure. Often, activities are executed with the goal of maintaining good relationships between sponsors and site staff, but the impact of these activities is difficult to measure. It may not be valuable to make a heavy investment in metrics for these activities if no definitive results or evidence of direct impact on recruitment can be satisfactorily measured (this does not mean that they should not take place, just that expectations need to be set for reporting outcomes).

The recruitment program needs to be planned to allow for fluctuations in tactic intensity so that impact can be measured. For example, if an online search engine spend is held constant over the duration of the program, it will be difficult to tease out impact on screening/enrollment. However, if the intensity level fluctuates, a correlation between higher/lower spends and higher/lower screening/enrollment rates may be seen. The same premise holds true for expending labor hours for tactics such as advocacy outreach and social media.

3. Identify Key Metrics for Each Goal.

Once the goals for each tactic have been established and prioritized, the key metrics to measure progress toward those goals can be identified. For example, if the overall program goal is to accelerate lagging enrollment, the metric of interest may be the change in accrual rate, expressed as patients per site, per month (p/s/m) from before to after the recruitment program. On the tactic level, if the goal is to educate patients about the study to increase the likelihood of their participation, a correlation between the use of patient communication tools and the rate with which interested patients agree to screen for the study would support a claim that patients who are more informed about the study are more likely to screen for it. In this case, the metric of interest would be the conversion rate from interested to screened.

Direct impact is difficult to measure for some tactics. In these cases, correlations between tactic execution and screening/enrollment rates can be measured. For example, if the study web site does not have a call to action that

Figure 2: Recruitment goal sample metrics

Recruitment goal	Metric
Build awareness in the physician community	• Awareness levels among relevant physicians
Communicating with patients about the study	• Conversion rate
	• Screen-fail rates
Building a referral network	• Size of or increase in referral network
	• Number of referrals
Increasing screenings	• Total number of screenings
	• Increase in screenings
Accelerating enrollment	• Accrual rate in p/s/m (patients per site, per month)
Meeting enrollment goals	• Total number of randomizations
	• Increase in randomizations

Source: MMG

can be tracked (e.g., the web site refers patients directly to investigative sites for follow up), the value of the web site could be measured indirectly by testing for a correlation of changes in overall screening/randomization activity during the time the site was active.

4. Define Success for Each Metric.

Once key metrics have been identified for every recruitment goal, success needs to be defined for each metric. For example, does an increase in referrals by 10 percent represent a successful referral networking effort? Does a boost in accrual rate from 0.75 p/s/m to 1.0 p/s/m indicate success for a $50,000 advertising campaign? The definition of success for individual metrics will vary from study to study depending on the particular challenges of a protocol. Success for one recruitment program could be increasing accrual by 10 percent, while an increase of 40 percent may be expected for another program. Again, this should be determined before the recruitment program begins so that all stakeholders understand not only the general goals (e.g., accelerate enrollment) but also the specific targets for each goal (e.g., increase accrual rate by 40 percent by date X).

It is important to be practical when determining what constitutes success. Referencing historical enrollment data for similar study scenarios and accounting fully for external, study-specific variables (e.g., incidence/prevalence data, current available treatment options and competing trials) will help stakeholders develop attainable goals.

5. Map Out All Required Data Points for Each Metric.

Like other data analysis exercises that require collection over time of multiple data points from multiple sources, recruitment performance data need formatting, scrubbing and quality checks. It is easy to underestimate the complexity of this effort or the time it may take to confirm that all required data points are accounted for, where they will come from, the timing for their collection, who will be responsible for ensuring they are collected and how they need to be formatted. The most common cause of holes in metrics analyses is that a data type or point was not identified for collection or the mechanism for its collection was not established. For example, Figure 3 describes the data needed to perform an accrual rate (p/s/m) comparison to measure the success of a two-week ad run without the support of a centralized call center for 20 sites in the U.S.

6. Set Up the Data Collection Processes.

Once all data points have been identified for each tactic, a detailed plan should be developed that outlines how and when they will be collected and who will be responsible for ensuring their collection. If data are being collected from sites, there must be a way to track completion status and a plan to

Figure 3: Necessary data for accrual rate comparison

Time point	Data points needed
Pre-tactic	• Date each site is open for enrollment
	• Date ad run starts for each of the 20 sites
	• If ad run is deployed after enrollment has begun, patient enrollment at each site with date of enrollment for each patient
	• If ad run is deployed after enrollment has begun, the current average screening-to-enrollment lag (to establish expected time to impact)
During/ post-tactic	• If reporting a screening-to-enrollment lag, expected impact date for each site
	• Date tactic-related results are expected to extinguish
	• Patients enrolled by site with enrollment date for each patient

Source: MMG

follow up on missing data with the same diligence as for the study data. Data collection workflows should be designed so that metrics data are collected in real time, rather than pieced together at the end of a program. From a performance management standpoint, real-time data collection and analysis enables program optimization, so that recruitment resources can be shifted to focus on the most effective tactics. It also is time-consuming to collect data retrospectively, particularly if it has not been captured in an easily accessible format.

7. Analysis and Reporting Plan.

Once the data collection process is established an analysis plan should be developed, much like a protocol's statistical analysis plan. An analysis plan for recruitment metrics should consider environmental factors such as seasonality, staff turnover at the sites and competing studies, which could affect the results. The plan should also include a test analysis using mock data to verify that the data collection mechanisms are in place, all required data points have been identified and the product of the analyses meets stakeholders' expectations.

Enlisting a third-party partner to help with the data analysis can greatly increase the perceived and actual validity of the analysis. It helps to remove bias that naturally and unconsciously becomes part of any data analysis. Using the same third-party partner across sets of studies increases cost efficiency and supports consistency.

The Next Generation of Global Recruitment Metrics

Recognition of centralized recruitment as a clinical trial management specialty and a way to gain significant cost efficiencies in the drug development life cycle has opened the gates to more strategic programs, pushed earlier recruitment planning and created a world in which recruitment metrics are not just possible, but expected. There is a growing expectation that proposed recruitment strategies are backed by metrics for relevant trials and not just by patient behaviors and motivations, the disease and competitive landscape and protocol-specific challenges levied on research sites.

As the industry builds a body of recruitment metrics that can be referenced, and as our collective understanding of enrollment influencers in given patient populations, regions and study types grows, we have the opportunity to apply predictive modeling to recruitment. Industry leaders are beginning to use scenario comparisons to weigh time and cost tradeoffs and to guide prioritizations as to which trials receive recruitment support and at what level. It is anticipated that this will help increase study teams' and sites' confidence in recruitment methodologies, which will allow their use to increase, contributing to a new generation of recruitment metrics the entire industry can leverage to benefit the most important stakeholders—the patients.

Author Biography

John has been the CEO of MMG, a global patient recruitment and retention firm, for the past six years. John has over 20 years of sales and sales management experience in healthcare, pharmaceutical and life science organizations. Prior to joining MMG, he managed business development teams at information technology (Hewlett Packard) and healthcare professional service provider organizations. At MMG, John's focus is measurable growth on revenue and profit while setting the vision for the company. He excels at creating partnerships—with vendors and within the pharmaceutical industry—that will bring measurable and cost-efficient results for clients. His passion for the work, inspiring his people and innovating in client service led him to be named one of the 100 most inspiring people by *PharmaVoice* magazine in 2006.

CHAPTER FIVE

Budgeting and Contracting for Global Recruitment and Retention Strategy: Site Considerations and ROW Implications

By Chris Trizna

As studies become more complex and patients harder to find, the importance of recruitment and retention of study participants has become increasingly critical. Developing a study budget has been more and more difficult with all of the different recruitment and retention needs and protocol complexity. There are many variables that must be considered in the protocol planning process.

But where do you start in building a budget? And, with the increase in Rest-Of-World (ROW) sites, how can you accurately budget for global studies? The patient recruitment landscape has changed dramatically over the past 10 years. One of the biggest changes is the number of studies in which ex-U.S. sites comprise the greatest percentage of study sites. These sites add a different level of intricacy to the budgeting and contracting process. Many different issues must be considered before budgeting for patient recruitment globally.

In this case study, an RFP for a major sponsor asked for pricing to enroll a large, 36-country, 300-site study. In the efforts to "simplify" the proposal process, vendors were asked to fill out a spreadsheet requiring costs for all countries using the same recruitment tactics.

Here are a few of the questions that were addressed before attempting to develop the budget for the RFP:

- When will the study begin?
- Have the sites been selected?
- How challenging is this protocol and finding the patients being sought?

- What is the enrollment timeline?
- How many patients will be needed from recruitment?
- Which countries are involved?
- Comparing cost with time, which is more important?

The following questions were pivotal to developing the RFP response:

1. *Have the sites been selected?*
   There are so many enrollment variables that depend on selecting the right sites. Recruitment strategy can change from one type of site to another. Is the site using a central or local IRB? Is the site located in a dense or populated area? What is the prevalence of the condition around the site? What is the economic and healthcare situation around the site? Utilizing multiple sites in the same area/markets can provide you with some potential budgeting efficiency.
2. *How challenging is this protocol and finding the patients being sought?*
   Today's protocols have made it much more difficult to find qualified subjects to enroll into a study. As an example, in years past recruiting patients for osteoarthritis studies was much different. New medications and treatments have been introduced that have lessened the need for some people to participate in studies. Studies have become more complex, with more inclusion/exclusion criteria and some requiring multiple conditions. The cost to recruit patients can vary widely, even within the same condition, based on the protocol design.
3. *What is the enrollment timeline?*
   The rate at which you need to enroll a study will depend greatly on where the patients are coming from. Given the right support and time, sites may be able to enroll patients from their private practice and not need to recruit from outside. It could take up to a year to get approval to start enrolling patients in some countries.
4. *How many patients will be needed from recruitment?*
   This is the number one variable for developing a budget! You will need to know how many patients are going to come from the site and how many are going to come from recruitment. The cost to recruit a patient from outside a practice is very expensive compared to one from within. Recruited patients also can be more expensive to retain. Every tactic will have a different cost to recruiting patients. The goal is to maximize the lowest cost tactics to keep you on budget and timeline.
5. *Which countries are involved?*
   Country selection is one of the most important questions to ask when considering a global study. The recruitment landscape changes annually and is completely different in every country. Ethics Board approvals can take up to one year in some countries, while the ability

to advertise in another country is prohibited. You will need to know which recruitment/retention tactics are available for use in order to build your budget.

6. *Comparing cost with time, which is more important?*
Both! But would it be worth $500,000 to finish a study three months ahead of schedule? How you manage the recruitment of a study can affect the timeline.

ROW considerations: Every country will have a different cost to acquire patients based on many different variables, which will be discussed throughout this chapter.

Preface to Developing a Recruitment Budget

Once these questions have been addressed, the first steps to determine methodology for budget development are in place.

One important question is: "Who are the patients we are looking for and where will we find them?"

There are three areas in which to locate participants:

1. Inside the practice or hospital
2. Within the community and referring physicians
3. Through external methods such as advertising

Recruitment Funnel

For each tactic a funnel will be required to be able to develop a budget. Building a funnel for each tactic will help identify not only the budget, but the resources needed. For example, if you need to generate 20 phone calls in order to screen four and enroll two, you may need to consider contracting with a call center to handle the high volume of calls.

In-Office Recruitment

You can locate patients within the physician practice in a number of ways. Identify them and reach out to them using IRB-approved materials. You also must be able to generate interest from those patients in your waiting room who have not been pre-identified. Patients enrolled within the practice will be your lowest-cost enrolled subjects.

As the study sponsor or CRO, there are a number of tools to consider developing for sites to use within their practices. Many recruitment companies bundle these tools into a Recruitment Kit or Box. It's important to make

Figure 1: Recruitment funnel

Funnel steps	Action	Variable
Total calls	Total calls generated	Media/Creatives/Chart reviews
Calls answered	Speaking with potential candidates	Ability to handle or make calls
Screening calls (60-70%)	Caller agrees to phone screening	Caller's interest in pursuing trial participation
Pre-qualify (10-60%)	Those who pre-qualify based on phone screening	Inclusion/Exclusion criteria
Show V1 (20-75%)	People who show up for screening	Individual's motivation
Medically screen (50-75%)	Consent to screening	Study coordinator effectively introducing study to subject
Consent and enroll (40-90%)	Meet I/E criteria	Medical I/E criteria screening

sure you are spending a little extra time and money creating professional and attractive tools. Including creative design and production, a typical recruitment kit will cost anywhere from $750 to $1,300 per site.

Some of the tools include:

- Patient brochures (100-500)
- Flyers (25-250)
- Easels (3-5)
- I/E Criteria pocket cards (3-5)
- Study buttons (3-5)
- Consent presentations (1-2)
- Chart flags (25-50)
- In-office study videos (1)
- Doctor to patient letters (electronic)
- Banners (1)

Each of these tools (and many others not mentioned here) can and will be used by each site differently.

ROW considerations: Remember, one creative may not support all countries in your study. If you are using people in your images, you may need new people who fit the demographics of other countries. Use of certain colors in different countries may need to be considered. The costs of translations, creative development, and approved tools need to be considered for ROW budget development.

Community-Based Recruitment

If you are able to recruit patients from outside the practice, developing recruitment tactics and tools to generate interest in the study from within the community can be an effective way to enroll patients.

This is an area in which many sites and study coordinators would like to focus more effort but don't have the time to develop the tools, build the community network and do the actual work. These tactics include physician outreach, health fairs, distributing study information to local organizations and pharmacies and Lunch and Learns.

Depending on the relevant tactics, their costs will vary. Typical tools needed for these tactics include:

- Patient brochures (250-1,000)
- Flyers (100-250)
- Easels (3-5)
- Banners (1)
- Doctor to doctor letters (electronic)
- Patient ID profile sheets for referring doctors (5)

ROW considerations: The healthcare situation is different in other countries than the United States. Outreach tactics will differ in each country. In some countries, all patients will be found within the office and there will be no need for physician outreach. In other countries, some of these tools are not allowed.

External Recruitment Through Advertising

When done correctly, media advertising can speed up the enrollment process and be cost efficient. When done incorrectly, it can be very expensive and frustrating. The traditional methods of advertising (or what I like to call direct response advertising) include television, radio, newspaper, direct mail and internet. Other recruitment tactics, described as "out of home" vehicles, include mass transit, billboards and movie theaters.

If you do not take the time and allocate the budget to develop professional and effective advertisements, you can cut your results in half, if not more.

I don't know how many times I have seen print ads created in Microsoft Word with clip art, or scripts that were approved for both radio and TV. Investing in professional creatives that capture your target audience's attention and gets them to go to a web site or make a phone call will pay huge dividends in your recruitment success. Developing your advertising messages at the beginning for all sites to use will minimize your development costs and maximize your recruitment results. Remember, sites typically do not employ graphic designers, media buyers or web developers—give them the support they need to be successful!

Building the Budget

The first thing is to determine your target audience and the best method to reach them via advertising. For example, you are not likely to use newspapers to target women ages 20 to 35 because they do not read the newspaper as much as they are online or listening to the radio. Selecting the most efficient media vehicle can increase response rates and enrollment by two to three times.

In creating a budget, you also need to know how many subjects you must recruit via advertising. Providing a site with a $2,000-$5,000 advertising budget may yield one or two subjects. If you need five or six subjects, you will need to provide the site with additional funds. Every condition will have a different cost to generate responses and enroll patients.

Figure 2: Average costs for three depression studies

Variables include the condition, inclusion/exclusion criteria included in the ad and the overall effectiveness of the ad itself.

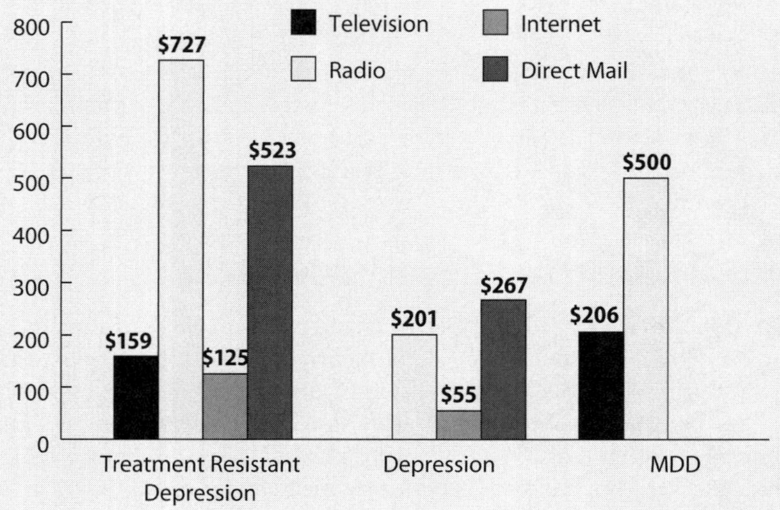

Source: Clinical Site Services

ROW considerations: Advertising outside of North America can be limiting. While countries are starting to loosen their advertising requirements, you will need to do a significant amount of research into which countries you can advertise and if it will be effective. Also, you will need to consider translation costs as well as the creative development process to match the customs and culture of each country. You can't simply translate a North American print ad and expect it to have the same impact, appeal and feeling when you place it in a foreign newspaper.

How Much Will You Need for Recruitment?

Without knowing where the patients will come from, how can you determine the cost of recruiting them? You should know how many patients will come from within the site's practice and how many will need to come from external avenues. The more patients a site can enroll from within its practice, the less costly recruitment will be. Here is an example of how a site may enroll subjects and how to develop a site budget.

Figure 3: How sites enroll

Source of enrollment	Percent	Number of patients
Internal	50%	5-7
Community	10%	1-2
External	40%	3-5
Goal total	100%	10

ROW considerations: First you must figure out what tactics and tools are approved for use. Second, you must budget for translations. Remember, there may be more than one language per country. Third, the cost to acquire a patient will vary in each country based on healthcare options, prevalence and patient populations.

Determining the Best Outsourcing Options

These are several different choices when selecting the best outsourcing scenario for your study. Each option needs to be weighed carefully in terms of how much control you want to have, your budget for these services and the aggressiveness of your study timeline.

1. **Full-service recruitment** companies can support your entire recruitment and retention program. These companies have historical information on the best tactics and response rates for different studies.

They provide a complete enrollment and retention strategy, have an in-house creative and media department and provide you with a call-handling solution, a team for site-support services and reporting on recruitment successes and consultation throughout your enrollment timeline.

Pros: Experience and metrics to provide budgets and best recruitment tactics, manages the entire process, provides you with reporting and consultation and can deliver centralized information easily and quickly shared with all sites.

Cons: High costs to manage the process, may lack individual attention for each specific site.

2. **Multiple point-of-contact recruitment vendors** are for those companies who want to manage the process but don't have the resources to execute recruitment. Companies to be considered include creative development companies, media buying companies, call centers, technology companies for web development and SMS capabilities and site support.

   Pros: Retain control to bring the best services together, manage the process yourself and minimize costs.

   Cons: Very labor intensive and difficult to coordinate, multiple project managers.

3. **Site-driven recruitment** activities put the responsibility for proper execution on each site. You would provide the tools to sites and let them develop and execute their own local campaigns.

   Pros: Much lower costs to run recruitment campaigns compared to centralized recruitment companies; typically, this is best when sites are confident they can recruit well within their practices with little or no advertising.

   Cons: If enrollment is behind, time is lost due to the outsourcing process during the study. Costs for rescue programs can be two to three times more expensive than prospective recruitment planning. There is little or no sharing of success (or failure) with different recruitment tactics.

Contract Options

In the past, few options existed for handling one's patient recruitment needs. If you were seeking recruitment help, you would hire a centralized patient recruitment company to take care of everything. A lot of money was spent developing these services and you were at the mercy of their pricing.

Today, many more options are available. There are more companies to choose from, providing more services with different contract alternatives. Depending on your needs, you can select companies to execute the services you require: creative development, production of print/video ads, media placement, call centers, web developers and recruitment management consultants.

There are different contracting methods available from which you can choose. The three most popular include:

1. Contract for Services (traditional)
2. Risk-Reward
3. Pay for Performance

Contract for Services is exactly what it means. The company will provide you the services you request. If you are managing the recruitment/retention program, you have control of what is done and the results.

Benefit: You know what you are paying for, and if you are managing the recruitment vendors you have the information to make good decisions and minimize the expense.

Downfall: Depending on how many different companies you are dealing with, it could get expensive and difficult to manage multiple vendors.

In a **Risk-Reward** contract, the vendor is risking some or all payments until a certain deliverable is met. In this type of contract, the vendor is going to want more control of the process to ensure goals are met. Typically, there is a huge benefit to the vendor if the goals are met or exceeded.

Benefit: If the vendor does not meet its goals, you do not pay for services not earned through expected performance.

Downfall: If the vendor does not meet its goals, you are still behind and will have to find a different solution. Vendors will also err on the high side of pricing to ensure they are going to make their goals, which could cost you more for enrollment services.

Pay for Performance is a new option in our industry. Basically, you pay for the results generated. In a traditional contract for hire, a recruitment company may charge you $500,000 for all services, including media, to enroll 200 patients. In a traditional contract, you would pay $500,000 even if your enrollment of 200 was not met. Pay for performance would divide the total cost by the number of enrolled, which would be $2,500 per patient.

Benefit: You pay for the number of patients enrolled with no risk of paying the total budget with no guarantees.

Downfall: The vendor will hedge its bets and probably charge much more per patient to make sure it covers costs, so the overall costs are much higher than if you contracted the traditional way. Also, there are typically many "out" clauses for the vendor; you still will have to pay the vendor for its out-of-pocket expenses. As with Risk-Reward contracts, if the vendor does not perform, you still need to find a solution but in a lot less time.

Retention

Retention and compliance is as important, if not more important, than recruitment. If you lose a patient during a study, you have to find a replacement—and in the meantime have lost valuable time and data. While there is an expense to retention, it typically is just a fraction of the cost to recruit. There are many methods of retaining and keeping subjects compliant with the protocol.

As with recruitment, retention is an activity that typically falls on the study coordinator. The challenge is that the coordinator doesn't have time to keep up with the activities needed to effectively retain subjects; this is important to keep in mind when developing a retention program.

Retention and compliance needs often include:

- **Study Visit Reminders**—These can usually be managed through phone calls, emails, SMS (texting), letters/post cards and appointment cards.

Figure 4 : Appointment reminder systems

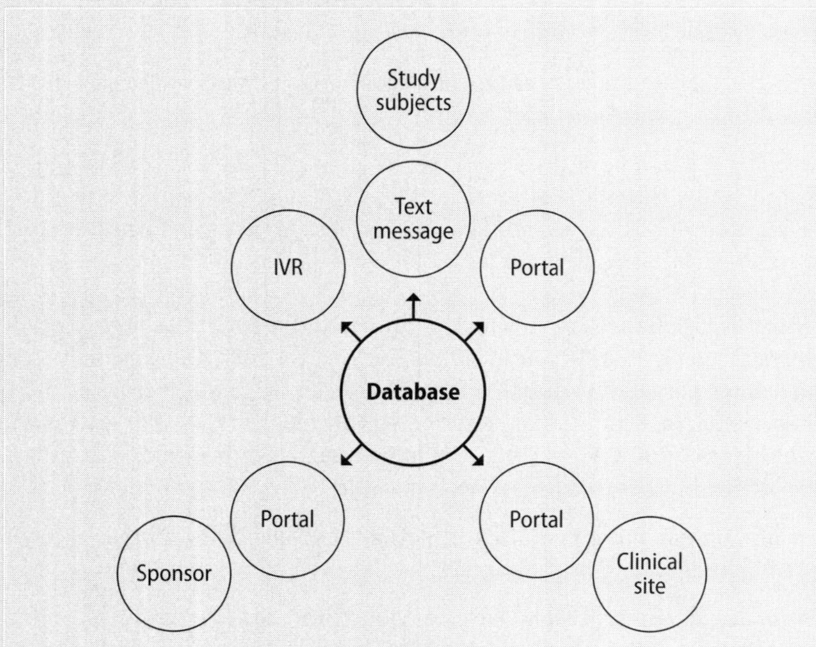

- **Participation Appreciation**—Show the subjects that you appreciate their time and recognize their commitment to the study. Gifts at each visit, personalized letters, educational materials and additional resources are good examples of showing appreciation.
- **Travel Support**—Time and travel expense can be a big challenge for some people. Budget for travel vouchers, bus or city transit cards or taxi services.
- **Compliance (dosing or diary) reminder**—This can be a challenge for some studies and their complicated processes. Providing calendars, phone calls, emails, SMS messages, alarm clocks or watches will increase the probability that patients will remain compliant.

With today's technology, there is no reason not to provide sites with appointment reminder support. There are systems patients opt into to be contacted by their preferred method, whether via phone call, email or text message. Systems also provide options to reschedule or respond to the study coordinator, and provide sponsors with metrics on retention rates. This takes a big burden off study coordinators and ensures the activity is completed.

ROW considerations: As with recruitment, you will have to check with the Ethics Boards of every country as to which tactics are approved for use. Translations and cost of production will affect the costs in each country.

Additional Variables

1. **Contingencies:** Who is to know what changes can potentially take place between the time of contracting and FPI? What if your study simply doesn't get the response you had hoped for? An unlimited number of situations can arise that have the ability to derail your study, or at least your budget. It is best to allow for a 10% contingency for any unplanned missteps.
2. **Site payments:** Are your payments to sites competitive with other studies? Sites are going to be less motivated to screen and enroll in your study if the incentive to do so is significantly less than that of another study.
3. **Protocol challenges:** Gone are the days of "simple" OA or T2D studies. Today's protocols more often than not are complex studies seeking difficult-to-reach populations. The complexity of the protocol will undoubtedly affect the funnel, which will increase the cost per enrolled patient.
4. **Country selection:** Smart country selection hopefully will alleviate the need for additional funds, but at times this is unavoidable. Match

prevalence/incidence rates of the therapeutic area with country selection will allow you to accomplish your goals in the most economical way possible.

5. **Global translations:** Any materials or messaging you have created for use in North America will need, at the very minimum, translations for use in other countries. You also may have to consider revising other elements of advertising materials, such as colors, images or fonts that could be offensive to people in certain countries.
6. **Ethics and approvals:** The approval processes outside North America vary greatly in terms of cost and timelines. Accounting for these costs is easier than calculating for site inactivity due to global approval timelines; you may need to utilize additional funds once these sites are active to recover lost time.
7. **Data protection in foreign countries:** Just like HIPAA regulations in the U.S., it is important to be aware of cost and timelines surrounding data privacy and protection. These will vary by country and depend on the extent of data captured.

Summary

Successfully planning and budgeting for patient recruitment requires significant insight, historical data and thoughtful preparation; adding global markets to the mix increases the level of complexity exponentially.

The intricacies of the protocol must be understood, and you must try to ascertain how each site will fare with internal recruitment. Timelines must be reviewed to determine if any external recruitment tactics need to be employed—and at what level and what point in the timeline. You'll face additional challenges if there are competitive studies or if site selection has left you with less-than-stellar sites. Lack of retention could increase your budget if dropout rates escalate and you need to recruit new patients.

Defining your contract and vendor needs early also will save you time and money, by allowing you to ask for exactly what you need in services, reporting and results. In determining the best outsourcing option for each study, you will have to weigh the importance of timeline versus cost.

Setting your study up for the best possible recruitment success can be achieved through thoughtful, strategic budgetary planning and smart contracting and outsourcing.

Author Biography

Chris Trizna is president of Clinical Site Services (CSS), which focuses on the patient recruitment sector by increasing site performance and optimizing patient enrollment. Chris founded CSS in 2005 with a mission to address the pharmaceutical industry's need for site-specific enrollment solutions. He provides sponsors, CROs, SMOs and investigative sites with strategic clinical trial consultation and directs patient enrollment services. In 2010 Chris co-founded CSSi (Clinical Site Services International), a global patient enrollment company with experience in more than 40 countries, concentrating on providing country-specific enrollment leadership. Chris is considered an industry thought leader and has presented at numerous conferences and meetings on the topic of patient enrollment. He has implemented more than 200 large-scale recruitment initiatives and has worked with many top pharmaceutical companies, CROs and SMOs, in addition to more than 2,000 sites. Chris received his Bachelor of Science in business administration from Virginia Commonwealth University. He is a member of ACRP and CISCRP.

CHAPTER SIX

Closing Enrollment Shortfalls in Centralized Patient Recruitment

By Richard Malcolm, Ph.D., Jill Pellegrino, Leah R. Garnett, Roger Smith and Joe O'Rourke

Optimizing Site Performance Through Additive Patient Enrollment

Twenty years ago, sites alone would provide the total enrollment for a study simply by reaching into their own databases of patients. But in the last two decades, the clinical trial landscape has changed; site enrollment is increasingly supplemented by patients sourced from outside of sites' own practices.

There are three main reasons for this change: 1) protocols have grown in complexity as a result of more stringent inclusion/exclusion criteria; 2) the number of patients required for clinical research is growing due to an increasing number of trials; and 3) There has been an increase in the number of patients required for each trial.

As a result, sites have had to screen larger numbers of patients from their practices to find even one randomized patient. The competition for patients at the sites has increased, and sites are exhausting their databases much faster. Today, sponsors are responding to these challenges by routinely using supplemental recruitment services to provide 30 percent to 50 percent or more of randomized subjects. For the majority of phase III trials , sites alone are unable to produce the entire enrollment needed and, more often than not, study teams are required to spend additional budget to supplement what the sites were expected do on their own.

Do You Really Know What You're Paying per Patient?

Many sponsors do not know what it costs to enroll each individual patient in a clinical trial, let alone what parts of the study budget to factor into the overall equation. It is imperative that study teams understand what they are paying on a per-patient, per-site basis to establish a baseline cost against which to evaluate their options.

A sponsor hires a site not simply for the facility, but for access to the pa-

Figure 1: The changing landscape of clinical trials

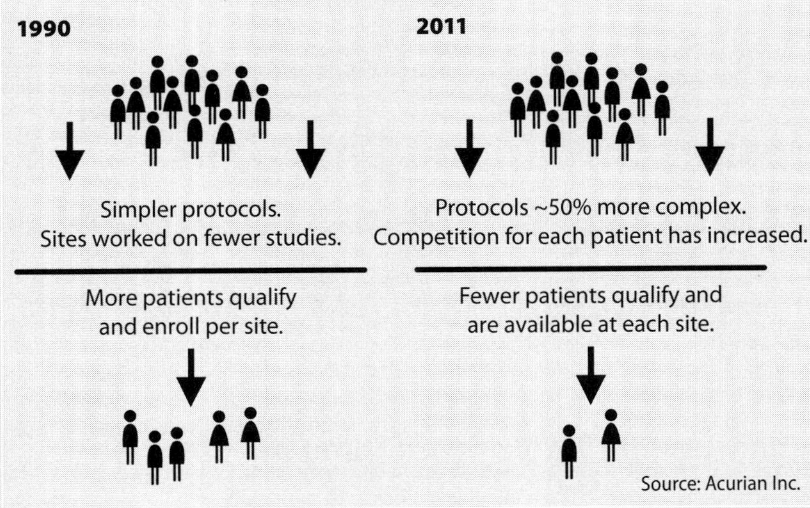

tients that site represents for the study. The cost of initiating a site is the down payment on those patients, regardless of how many patients the site ends up contributing. Study teams determine the number of sites they need based on the average number of patients they expect each site to recruit. Whenever possible, study teams seek to minimize the number of sites.

This is because **more sites** = **higher study costs.**

More patients recruited per site = **fewer study sites** = **lower study costs.**

Once you know the average number of patients needed per site, the cost per patient can be calculated by dividing the cost of initiating the average site by the number of patients you expect to yield from the average site.

Therefore:

$$\frac{\text{Cost of initiating a site}}{\text{Expected number of patients}} = \text{Site cost per patient}$$

Estimates from Cutting Edge Information, a pharmaceutical business intelligence firm, put the cost of initiating a site at $20,000 to $75,000. Assume each site will cost an average of $25,000 to hire, train and prepare to see patients. Now assume each site will contribute an average of five patients. The study team is paying $5,000 per patient from a site.

Conducting this exercise successfully benchmarks the current base cost for each patient "recruited" from investigators, assuming the investigators recruit all the patients required to close enrollment. However, since sites can no longer shoulder 100 percent of the enrollment burden, they will not provide the average number of patients sponsors expect and, therefore, cost per patient will increase.

If patient enrollment costs are estimated at $5,000 per patient based on a site contributing five enrolled patients against initiation costs of $25,000, the cost per patient will rise as the number of patients contributed declines, because the site initiation costs are fixed, regardless of site performance.

In the scenario above:

- If a site contributed 3.75 patients, requiring 25 percent of enrollment from sources outside the site, the cost per patient would be $6,667.
- If a site contributed 2.5 patients, requiring 50 percent of enrollment from sources outside the site, the cost per patient would be $10,000.

It is important to note that these numbers do not include additional recruitment monies expended for local recruitment support, such as site stipends, which are often $2,500 to $5,000.

Once a study team concludes that sites alone will not meet their enrollment needs in time, limited choices are available to make up the patient gap. All of the choices cost money and have varying time implications. Therefore, the study team must ask, "What is the most cost-effective way to obtain the patients we need, within the timeframe we need and at the lowest risk of failure?" Now is the time to assess where sponsors can get the most value, whichever option they choose.

Limited Options for Fixing Enrollment Issues

The most common choices for making up patient shortfalls include:

1. **Add more sites:** This often means more cost and time, and no guarantee of site performance.
2. **Do nothing and wait:** This often means spending money on study operations while enrollment is at a standstill. This is an expensive delay of the inevitable need to spend money to get enrollment back on track.
3. **Give sites money for local advertising:** This means untracked expenditures, no accountability and no guarantee of results.
4. **Hire recruitment support based on results:** This means you pay only for results—patient commitments are aligned to financial interests.

The following points assist in assessing the typical impact of each one on time, budget and enrollment effectiveness.

1. Add More Sites.

When the top sites the sponsor has selected fall short on their numbers, there is little chance that adding second- or third-tier sites will match or do better than either the highest performing sites or those with more robust patient populations. Additionally, it takes months and great expense for a sponsor or CRO to add sites to an ongoing study. Adding sites can cost from $20,000 to $75,000 per site.

2. Do Nothing and Wait.

Sites are small businesses. Sponsors hire them to provide patients per a negotiated contract. This is revenue a site needs to pay expenses and realize a profit, so it is not holding out when it comes to enrolling patients. If sites are not finding patients now, they will not suddenly produce them in a few weeks. And as a sponsor waits for the magic, the study budget continues to dwindle. Sites still need to be monitored, IVRS is still running, drug supply is expiring, etc. Doing nothing has a substantial cost.

3. Give Money to Sites for Local Advertising.

Providing $2,500 to $5,000 to each site for local advertising is a long-standing practice, if not tradition. Yet the efficacy of providing local advertising stipends to sites is questionable. Some sites do a good job spending their advertising stipends efficiently, but most do not, and will be the first to admit it. Additionally, there is limited tracking of how sites spend these dollars and what results from their efforts. How can a sponsor know that the money it allocated was specifically spent on? How many enrolled/randomized patients were received for the stipend? Was the money spent recruiting patients who were directed to its study (versus a competing one)?

Such a lack of accountability is unacceptable in any other area of study management or an organization. The bottom line is that individual study sites are not experts in advertising or media buying; they are experts in patient care.

4. Develop an Organized, Sophisticated Recruitment Plan Based on Results.

Hiring a specialty vendor to design and manage an additive recruitment campaign focused on enhancing individual site enrollment makes the best sense from a time, risk and financial standpoint. However, the call to action is not to simply specialize in patient recruitment advertising.

Advertising is a component of patient recruitment, but patient recruitment is not advertising. Advertising agencies do advertising. Companies with a true expertise in patient recruitment use a set of proven processes in which recruitment is managed from the moment a patient responds to an advertisement through his or her initial eligibility pre-screening, first visit to the site, review of consent and ultimate enrollment in the study.

On the most basic level, pharmaceutical companies are the experts in drug development, sites are the experts in patient care, CROs are the experts in study conduct and true patient recruitment companies are the experts in recruiting, enrolling and retaining patients. Patient recruitment is a critical part of a study's success, and it needs to be managed by a company that specializes in it.

This central management of recruitment, enrollment and retention is de-

Figure 2: Value: Roles and expertise

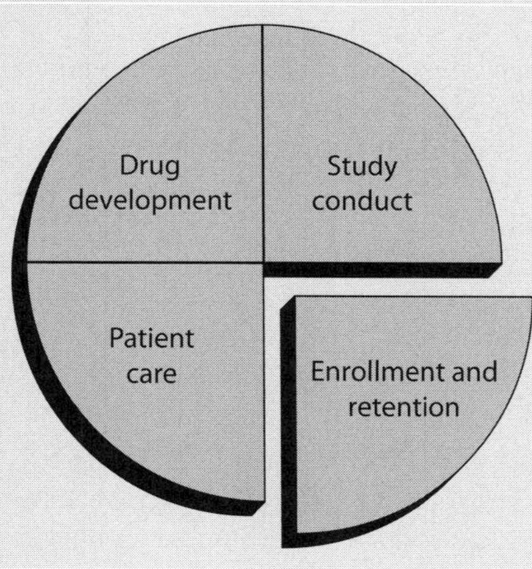

Source: Acurian Inc.

signed to optimize the performance of every site. These processes use the raw material created by many different forms of advertising to ensure that, with the help of each site, potential patients are managed and enrolled in the most timely and cost-efficient manner. A central recruitment campaign should ensure that sites always have a steady supply of additive, suitable patients to screen; these are patients sites otherwise would not have enrolled in the study because they are not part of the sites' existing databases.

Ask the recruitment provider if its contribution is predictable in terms of number of patients enrolled over a specific period of time. The partner also should be able to offer a fee structure based on the delivery of enrolled/randomized patients depending on the therapeutic area. That per-patient fee often can include all setup, project management and pass-through fees.

Sites are hired to contribute a certain number of patients; a centralized recruitment campaign should fill the gap, not provide ambiguous support. A recruitment partner confident in its assessment of enrollment challenges will contractually put the vast majority of its fees on the delivery of patients into the study.

And those patients should not be ones who would have been found through the sites' own activities. A recruitment partner should be confident that independent controls (site feedback, IVRS-data matching) will verify that those patients came into the study only as a result of the partner's work.

How Existing Site Contracts Disincentivize Success

As trials require a larger and larger share of their enrollment from sources outside of the investigator's practice, sites now serve two distinct recruitment roles: They are sources of patients, in that they enroll patients from within their own practices, and they act as a point of processing for patients from outside sources. Although this is a major paradigm shift, site contracts and relationships are still managed as if all of the enrolled patients come from inside the practices. Although sponsors now recognize that sites cannot always find patients on their own and additive recruitment has become a necessary part of enrolling trials, the study contracts have not reflected this new workload dynamic. In other words, as additive recruitment campaigns have dramatically increased the number of referrals sent to sites, there has been no change in the way sites are reimbursed for processing these patients.

Efficient processing of additive patients requires staff, a sense of urgency, persistence and significant administrative work to validate the quality of the potential volunteers prior to in-office evaluation. However, site contracts are currently set up to compensate post-consent, which assumes the patients were readily available from the sites' own practices. This misalignment in compensation causes waste in the form of patients left behind. When the names of qualified referrals are sent to the sites by an additive recruitment company, but these patients are never contacted, interviewed and scheduled, this radically increases the cost per randomization.

For example, a complex protocol that may require sites to process externally referred patients represents an eight-fold increase over what the sites normally see when they recruit patients on their own. Figure 3 demonstrates the difference in workload for a site processing in-practice patients versus externally referred patients.

Contacting, evaluating and processing each new patient takes time and resources. If sites are paid only for screening and enrollment and not for the

Figure 3: Workload difference between investigator database and central recruitment

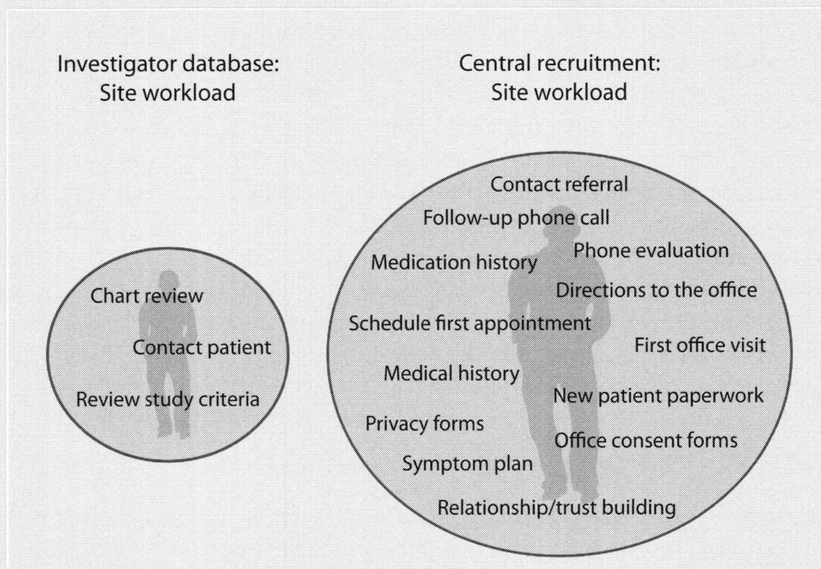

Source: Acurian Inc.

upstream, or pre-consent, work of interacting with potential patients, many sites cannot devote the resources necessary to make additive recruitment as efficient as it can be.

Differences in Site Performance

Here is a real-life example of how a lack of incentive by sites to screen patients changes the price per enrolled patient. A top 20 pharma company was running a phase III Major Depressive Disorder (MDD) trial across 45 U.S. sites. Due to an unexpected increase in screen-failure ratio, the sites were unable to meet the enrollment goal from their own patients. Therefore, the sponsor hired a recruitment vendor to supply additive patients to fill the enrollment gap. Over five months, the recruitment vendor sent the 45 sites a total of 1,882 pre-screened referred patients. From the 1,882 referred patients, the sites were able to screen 390, or 21 percent.

However, when the number of screened patients was analyzed across the sites, a vast difference in performance was noted. To assess the differences in performance across sites, the sites were grouped into four equal tiers based on the ratio of screened patients to pre-screened referrals. Tier 1 represents the top-performing sites and Tier 4 represents the bottom-performing sites. Each tier consists of the same number of sites and relatively the same number of pre-screened referrals. Each pre-screened referral took the identical screener; therefore, there was no difference in quality of the pre-screened referrals among the four groups of sites. Lastly, the sites in each group are spread throughout the country and are not heavily concentrated in any geographic area within each tier.

As Figure 4 demonstrates, the sites in Tier 1 were able to collectively screen 175 of the 421 pre-screened referrals they received, or 42 percent. The 12 sites in Tier 4 were able to collectively screen only 19 of the 494 pre-screened referrals they received, or 4 percent. A good number of the 12 sites in Tier 4 screened zero patients.

Cost Implications

A difference of 42 percent screened patients versus 4 percent screened patients has cost implications for the sponsor. Figure 5 demonstrates the difference in cost per screened patient for each tier. Each of the 175 patients screened at the Tier 1 sites cost $1,222 to secure. Each of the 19 patients screened at the Tier 4 sites cost $13,208 to secure. In other words, because some sites did not have the time or incentive to screen the qualified referrals they received, the referrals were simply 'lost.' Money was spent to recruit and screen them, but they were never contacted. This drives up the cost of recruiting all of the study's patients.

The study's overall cost per screened patient was $2,451; however, if all sites were incentivized to screen at the same rate as the Tier 1 sites, the overall cost per screened patient would have been $1,222, saving the sponsor a total of $479,310 (380 screened patients at $2,451 each, versus 380 screened patients at $1,122 each).

Figure 4: Site performance across tiers within an MDD study

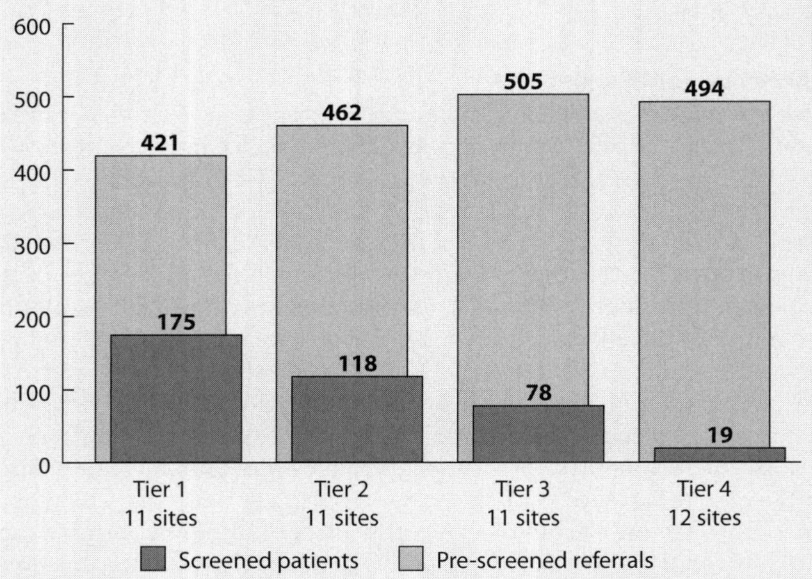

Source: Acurian Recruitment Manager database

Revisiting Site Contracts

Sites are, for the most part, small businesses. They have standard operation issues (cash flow, resource management, etc.) and will make rational decisions based on revenue and cost. If sites continue to be put into the unfair position of 'processing' external patients needed to close enrollment without being paid to do the work, they will not and, they could argue, should not, do the work. Clearly, old site contracts have not kept up with the present-day reality: Up to 50 percent of all clinical trials are filled through central recruitment, but site contracts reflect the days when sites enrolled patients on their own. Sifting through externally referred patients takes time, urgency and focus. The successful sites are those that "put in the work."

The cost of reimbursing a site's processing work is minuscule compared to the cost of waste in unachieved enrollment. The difference in price per patient in the MDD scenario is dramatic: $1,222 at one site versus $13,208 at another. It doesn't have to be this way. It is time to acknowledge that the landscape has changed, and that additive recruitment is a necessary component of successful and timely enrollment and, as such, requires its own reimbursement paradigm that reflects the different levels of work at different parts of the recruitment process. When sponsors revise site contracts to properly compensate sites for processing externally recruited and referred patients, the costs of external patient recruitment will dramatically decrease.

Figure 5: Cost per screened patient across tiers within an MDD study

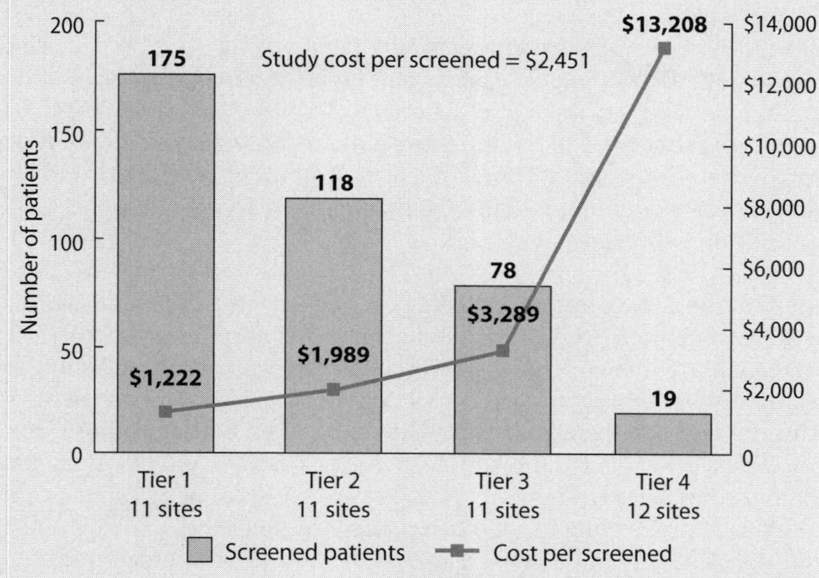

Source: Acurian Recruitment Manager database

Author Biographies

Richard "Rick" Malcolm, Ph.D., Chief Executive Officer of Acurian, brings more than 22 years of experience in healthcare management to his role. Previously, Rick was vice president, business development for global CRO Icon Clinical Research. Rick began his career in healthcare at SmithKline Beecham Pharmaceuticals (now GlaxoSmithKline), where he was responsible for product marketing of several cardiovascular, gastrointestinal, depression and anti-arthritic products. In addition to serving as worldwide head for SBCL's Clinical Trials Center (now Quest's central laboratory), he has held senior management and consulting roles at start-up pharmaceutical companies including The Medicines Company and Neutris Pharmaceuticals. Rick received his B.S. in Microbiology at the University of Michigan and his Ph.D. in Pharmacology at the University of Southern California.

Jill Pellegrino is director of recruitment strategy and analytics at Acurian, where she heads project feasibility and predictive modeling. Previously, she was head statistical analyst in Radian Guaranty's Risk Management department. Jill holds a B.A. in mathematics from LaSalle University.

Leah R. Garnett is a recruitment strategist at Acurian, where she focuses on feasibility analysis, patient motivation and outreach strategy for clinical trials. She is former editor of the Harvard Health Letter and a former senior web editor for The Children's Hospital of Philadelphia.

Roger Smith is Senior Vice President of Operations for Acurian. He brings more than 12 years of senior management experience in operations, product development and technology to his role at Acurian. Previously, Roger was Senior Vice President, Chief Information Officer for Kozmo.com; Vice President, Internet Strategy and Development at Petopia.com (PETCO); and Vice President, Programming at Sony Online Ventures, Inc. Roger holds a B.S. from Boston University.

Joe O'Rourke designs and develops customized patient enrollment solutions for Acurian's customers, bringing eight years of clinical research experience in patient enrollment operations, project delivery, patient care and study execution. He has managed over 40 recruitment campaigns at Acurian across a diverse array of therapeutic areas. Previously, he held positions within project delivery at United BioSource Corp., at Chester County Hospital providing cardiology care and as a research assistant at Johns Hopkins School of Medicine performing metabolic research. Joe holds a B.S. in kinesiology from West Chester University and an M.B.A. from Villanova University.

CHAPTER SEVEN

New Opportunities and Ethical Principles in Creative Design for Recruitment and Retention Materials

By Felicia Fuller and Diana L. Anderson-Foster, Ph.D.

Every study needs a voice that communicates the clinical trial sponsor's core objectives. Skilled patient recruitment professionals provide this through compelling messages and artful designs that resonate with target audiences and inspire study participation. As a key component of a recruitment and retention campaign, study collateral must be current, compelling and regulatory-compliant to achieve the sponsor's goals. Among these features the latter is most essential, to ensure legal acceptance and patient comprehension. To that end, clinical research professionals must consider literacy and all its facets when developing health materials and communication strategies for a range of diverse audiences—each with differing abilities, experiences and expectations.

Effective patient and physician-facing content is developed with facts, not fluff, so the research must be sound. Following client consultation, every assignment should get underway with thorough review of the protocol and in-depth research of the disease indication and target audience. From the etymology of words in messaging to the cultural connotation of color in designs, efforts in the research realm inspire accurate and targeted campaigns.

Creating Collateral with Health Literacy in Mind

According to Healthy People 2020, a U.S. health promotion and disease prevention initiative, an individual is considered to be "health literate" when he or she possesses the skills to understand information and services and use them to make appropriate decisions about health.

Health literacy incorporates a range of abilities: to read, comprehend and analyze information; to decode instructions, symbols, charts and diagrams; to weigh risks and benefits; and, ultimately, to make decisions and take action. However, the concept of health literacy extends to the materials, environments and challenges specifically associated with disease prevention and health promotion, including:[1]

- Patient-physician communication
- Drug labeling and medical instructions
- Health publications and other resources
- Informed consent document
- Medical and insurance forms
- Patient history
- Public health training
- Assessments for allied professional programs such as social work

Healthy People 2020 outlines key points for achieving health literacy, stating that it is fundamental to reducing health disparities. Two key areas are emphasized as crucial to attaining measurable improvement:

1. Develop appropriate written materials for audiences with limited literacy.
   - Health communicators should use existing resources to create plain language health communications targeted to this population.
   - Professional publications and federal documents already provide the necessary criteria.
2. Improve the reading skills of persons with limited literacy.
   - Health literacy programs can be tailored to target skill improvement.
   - These programs could be offered through a variety of organizations, such as libraries, schools and community groups.

Assessing Readability

Readability describes the ease with which a document can be read. A number of readability tests have been developed to assess the suitability of documents. These tests are based on mathematical formulas that correlate measurable elements of writing, such as the number of personal pronouns in the text, the average number of syllables in words or the number of words per sentence. The results of these tests depict the readability of the document in terms of grade levels according to the U.S. educational system (e.g., third grade, sixth grade).

It is important to note that not all features that promote readability can be measured mathematically (such as format and content). Nor can the mathematical equations measure comprehension directly. Nonetheless, the formulas are considered to be predictions of reading ease and provide some insight into how well the reader will understand ideas presented in the text.

A number of formulas, manual and electronic, can be used to evaluate readability. Regardless of the method, the formulas are usually based on one semantic factor and one syntactic factor. Semantic factors relate to the difficulty of words, whereas syntactic factors relate to the difficulty of sentences. Words are measured either against a frequency list or according to their length of characters or syllables. Sentences are measured for the average length of characters or words.

Most word processing software programs provide several readability measures. Microsoft Word offers many readability statistics. This function is found under "Options" in the "Tools" menu bar. Under the "Spelling and Grammar" tab is a check box marked "Show Readability Statistics." If this box is checked, Word automatically will display a summary of the readability after conducting a spell-check of the document.

The FOG Index is calculated by dividing the total number of words by the total number of sentences to equal (1) the average number of words per sentence. The number of words with more than three syllables is divided by the total number of words to equal the percentage of difficult words (2). Total figures (1) and (2) and multiply that total by 0.4 (3). This figure (3) is the FOG Index in years of education.

The SMOG Grading Formula uses three passages of 10 sentences, each from the beginning, middle and end of the document. Or, if the text has fewer than 30 sentences, all are included. The reading level is a function only of the number of polysyllabic words (words with three or more syllables) in the sampled text, with more polysyllabic words corresponding to higher reading levels. This formula is widely used and the National Cancer Institute has adopted it as the preferred method for assessing the readability of patient communications.

SMOG = 3 + the square root of (PSC) where PSC is the average polysyllable count per 10 sentences.

Figure 1: SMOG example

	Number of polysyllabic words in 10 consecutive sentences
Beginning	14
Middle	10
End of document	24
Average PSC Count	16
The square root of 16=	fourth-grade reading level

The Fry Readability Graph (FRG) has been validated for both Spanish and English-language documents. The FRG uses three sample passages of text, each exactly 100 words in length, from the beginning, middle and end of the source document. The grade level is computed as a function of the number of sentences and words contained in the three samples of text.

Improving Readability of Patient Educational Materials

Numerous techniques can be used to simplify the language and presentation of information in patient educational materials. The Centers for Disease Control and Prevention (CDC) offers several guidance documents for enhancing the readability of informed consent documents.[2] Some of the key suggestions for lowering the reading level include:

- Write patient-directed content on a 6th-to-8th-grade reading level; however, do not make assumptions about people who read at a low level. Maintain an adult perspective.
- Focus on a few key concepts.
- Structure content logically. Some patients prefer step-by-step instructions, while others may find concepts arranged from the general to the specific easier to understand.
- Find alternatives for complex words, medical jargon, abbreviations and acronyms. When no alternatives are available, spell out complex terms and abbreviations phonetically and give clear definitions.
- Keep most sentences short (16-word maximum, in most cases). Use varied sentence lengths to make them interesting, but keep sentences simple.
- Use active voice instead of passive voice where culturally acceptable.
    - For example:
      Active: Each study participant should use his or her inhaler daily.
      Passive: The inhaler should be used by study participants daily.
    - Consider, however, that in cultures such as Japan and China, active voice is viewed as condescending and rude. Conversely, in other countries—including the U.S.—passive voice is often viewed as awkward and indirect. For guidance, read material written in English for and by people in the country in question and make note of whether they prefer active or passive voice. Adjust your writing accordingly. When in doubt, use active voice. It is generally better understood by non-native English speakers.
- Be consistent with terms. For example, do not use "drugs" and "medications" interchangeably in the same document.

- When possible, say things positively, not negatively. For example, say "Record medication responses in your patient diary" instead of "Don't forget to record medication responses in your diary."
- Avoid slashes (e.g., he/she) because the reader may have trouble knowing if you mean both, or one or the other.
- Avoid false subjects by starting sentences with "It is" or "There are." What is "it" or "there" referring to? Here are a few examples:
  - It is required to follow medication schedule.
    Better to say: Medication compliance is required.
  - There are stickers on the patient calendar denoting your study visits.
    Better to say: Stickers on the patient calendar denote your study visits.
- Avoid double negatives. In English, a phrase like "not unpleasant" means "pleasant" (or at least "tolerable"), but in other languages, double negatives are interpreted differently and could be interpreted as "extremely unpleasant."
- Label any references to currency. You probably won't list sums of money in currencies for more than one or two countries, but do name whichever currency you list. Remember that the dollar sign ($) denotes currencies in various countries, so indicate which country is intended, e.g. USD, AUD.
- Write out dates. The ways in which dates are written can vary from country to country. For example, 6/2/12 can mean February 6 or June 2.
- List quantities in metric units. Only three nations in the world do not officially use the metric system: Myanmar, Liberia and the U.S. If you are not using the metric system, and you want your work to reach a global audience, it is time to start. This applies to distances, ingredient amounts, height, weight, etc.
- Keep in mind that while most countries officially use the metric system, some of them continue to use Imperial units. If your writing is aimed at readers in the U.K., for example, you might indicate weight not only in kilograms, but also in stone.

Colors and Symbols

The cultural connotations of colors and symbols vary widely, so it is prudent to thoroughly research historical perceptions to ensure the graphic elements of your communication pieces convey the appropriate messages. In most of Europe and the Americas, for example, white is associated with purity and marriage. However, in Japan, China and parts of Africa, white is traditionally the color of mourning.

Other rudiments of graphic design: Ensure images of people in patient-directed materials are consistent with the study population. For example, materials aimed at patients with sickle cell anemia, a disease that disproportionately affects individuals of African descent, should not depict Caucasians. Additionally, it is ill-advised to feature images of people who appear markedly healthier than the target population (e.g., a multiple sclerosis advertisement that features a subject mountain climbing). Lastly, keep captions close to graphics; avoid graphs and charts unless they aid understanding; balance the use of text, graphics and clear or "white" space; and avoid using words in all capital letters unless they are true acronyms.

Choosing a Translation Provider

As clinical trials continue their current path of global expansion, translation services have risen in the ranks as an essential selling point. Yet all translation companies are not created equal. Before hiring linguists to translate your clinical trial materials, ask the following key questions:

1. **Where are your translators based?** Many companies outsource translation services to countries in which labor is cheap and workers are poorly trained. Conversely, others hire U.S.-based translators who are not native speakers and lack understanding of colloquialisms and cultural connotations. Do not take the risk of your translations missing the mark—or worse—offending your intended audience.
2. **Are your translators generalists or industry specialists?** Linguists do more than convert words from one language to another. Any translation software can do that. Professional translators also convey concepts and ideas and, therefore, must be proficient in the subject at hand. With the complexity of technical concepts and regulatory requirements for patient communication, translating for the life sciences requires a level of skill not found among generalists.
3. **Is your translation provider certified?** International Organization for Standardization (ISO) certification is a designation reserved only for translation providers meeting the highest global standards. Certification is a rigorous process involving third-party assessment of company processes and procedures, including quality control, record keeping and client communication. It typically takes more than a year to complete. There are other certification programs similar to ISO, so do your homework.

Practical Application of Creative Collateral

A multidimensional patient recruitment strategy is required to compete globally amid changing industry dynamics. A program's viability is determined by its ability to captivate and inform the target audience; meet regulatory standards governing patient communication; and allow for accurate tracking, monitoring and metric reporting. Global recruitment programs must be developed with an understanding that external initiatives may be less relevant or appropriate in densely populated regions with specialized healthcare institutions than in other areas where patient access is more restrictive due to geographic spread or competing trials. For these regions, tools and materials developed to facilitate patient identification within individual institutions are more appropriate than public awareness-building campaigns. For example, U.S. strategies often include social media and direct-to-patient advertising, whereas, ROW initiatives emphasize physician education and site support. Below are examples of various recruitment program components:[3]

Site Support Materials

- Designed to aid sites in identifying and screening patients for trial participation
- Components include pocket protocols, inclusion/exclusion booklets or cards, study flowcharts, pre-screening worksheets and informed consent flipcharts
- Study flowcharts and inclusion/exclusion booklets and cards may have the most utility for sites

100% of sites surveyed said site support materials are useful for identifying and screening patients. (Rheumatoid Arthritis study)

Community Outreach

- Fosters study awareness among patients not currently known to sites
- May include speaking, exhibiting or participating in special events, fundraisers and health fairs
- Targets are associations and support groups as well as community clinics

95% of global sites surveyed said community outreach is effective for identifying trial participants. (Diabetes study)

Physician Education Packages

- Provide potential referring physicians with study details required to refer their patients for trial participation
- May include a physician-to-physician letter, physician brochure, inclusion/exclusion reference card and study-branded folder
- Sent to physicians who see patients with diabetes in close proximity to sites

95% of global sites consider physician education packages an effective recruitment strategy. (Cardiovascular Disease study)

Direct-to-Patient Advertising

- Patients frequently self-identify in response to targeted media campaigns
- Mixed-media program may include print, radio, television, social media and pay-per-click advertising on top internet search engines
- Pre-screener layered into study web site
- Effectiveness measured via performance analysis and metrics reporting

Only **42%** of global diabetes sites reported having previously used patient advertising.

Securing Site Commitment for Program Success

Achieving enrollment success lies in clinical trial sponsors' understanding that patient recruitment and retention strategies are only as effective as the sites commissioned to implement the plans. By aggressively educating and engaging sites, sponsors can mitigate competitive challenges, maintain statistical advantage and realize enrollment success. Central to this effort are 1) identifying high-performing sites equipped to execute program plans, 2) training clinical staff in recruitment fundamentals and 3) motivating sites throughout enrollment. Yet, before any of these steps can occur, the trial sponsor must be fully educated about, invested in and committed to the strategy. After all, though responsibility for execution is shared, the onus of outcome rests squarely with the sponsor as program progenitor and enforcer.

Author Biographies

Felicia Fuller is Publications Manager for DAC Patient Recruitment Services, an Imperial company, leading the editorial development of all client and corporate promotional collateral including print, broadcast and online content targeted to clinical and lay audiences. She is a published writer with 19 years of experience in multiple industries, having worked as a newspaper reporter, magazine editor and corporate publications strategist. Felicia won a 2011 Hermes Award for the article, "A Question of Color: Overcoming Barriers to Minority Research Participation."

Over a career spanning more than 25 years, Diana L. Anderson-Foster, Ph.D., has helped pioneer best practices in patient recruitment and retention for global clinical trials—first as founder, president and CEO of D. Anderson & Company and today as president of DAC Patient Recruitment Services, an Imperial company. Her book credits include *International Patient Re-*

cruitment: Regulatory Guidelines, Customs and Practices; A Guide to Patient Recruitment; and A Guide to Patient Recruitment and Retention. In 2006, PharmaVOICE named her among the 100 Most Inspiring People in the Life Sciences Industry. She also received an International Women of Influence Award from the Global EXEC Women's International Council in 2008, among other honors.

References

1. Healthy People 2020
2. Consent for CDC Research—A Reference for Developing Consent Forms and Oral Scripts
3. DAC Patient Recruitment Services

CHAPTER EIGHT

Social Networking and Technological Influences on Recruitment and Retention Strategy

By Kristy Wort

Social media has redefined the rules of marketing like no other medium in recent times. From tweeting about corporate accomplishments and friending industry colleagues on Facebook to seeking or posting job opportunities on LinkedIn, social media has revolutionized the way businesses communicate with internal and external audiences.

According to the 2011 Social Media Marketing Industry Report sponsored by Social Media Examiner, 93% of businesses are employing social media tactics to support their marketing strategies. Specifically, pharmaceutical companies increasingly leverage social media to promote clinical trial opportunities and engage prospective participants. Since February 2010, the number of individuals using social media in the United States has grown from roughly 115 million to 149 million, and from 244.2 million to 314.5 million abroad.[1]

The top four tools used by marketers are Facebook, Twitter, LinkedIn and blogs.[2]

The Role of Social Media in Clinical Trial Recruitment

Enrollment delays cost pharmaceutical companies $8 million each day a study is delayed, according to a recent report from Cutting Edge Information. These delays are normally due to recruiting patients into the trial. According to the Center for Information and Study on Clinical Research Participation, missed enrollment deadlines extend phase I studies by 42% on average, while phase II and III studies last 31% and 30% longer, respectively.[3]

To enroll clinical trials more quickly, the general public must become aware of specific opportunities, eligibility criteria, goals of the research and their protections as participants. According to an article in *Nature Biotech-*

Figure 1: Commonly used social media tools

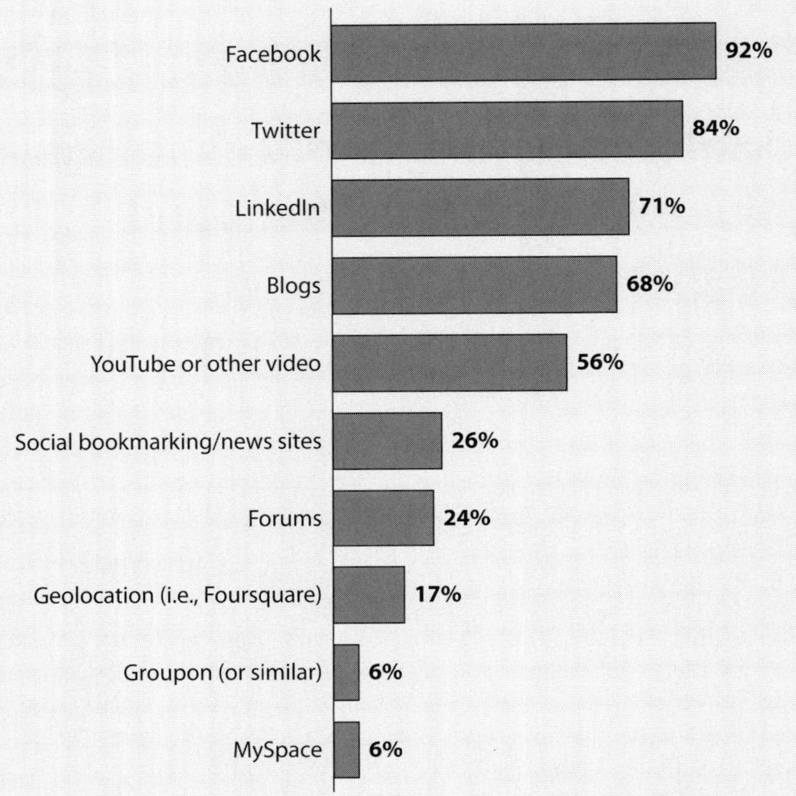

Source: 2011 Social Media Marketing Industry Report

nology, 94% of the public realizes the potential their participation could have on the advancement of medical science. Yet 75% of the general public states they have little or no knowledge about current opportunities and what they need to do to participate.[4]

To raise study awareness, a variety of tools may be deployed. Site-focused recruitment materials can be placed in the most prominent locations for potential study patients' viewing. These might include a site's reception area or a referring physician's office reception area. Community outreach is another effective way to reach potential patients. This is especially true in certain indications such as diabetes and multiple sclerosis, for which the support and advocacy community is active and close-knit. Building study awareness within the medical community also can generate interest and referrals from physician colleagues. Physician-to-physician materials that include a letter, fliers and brochures have proven effective in educating physicians and other healthcare practitioners about study opportunities.

Based on experience recruiting for difficult patient populations, social media is a new strategy to complement a multimedia campaign, but don't expect to completely enroll a study from it. Having a Facebook page is not considered social media in patient recruitment, since technically there is no ongoing interaction. It's impossible to control what is being posted, and although this can be monitored on a regular basis, it can't be 24/7. Utilizing pay-per-click advertising on Facebook has been extremely inexpensive in terms of overall cost. The challenge, as with all traditional media, is ensuring a clear, concise call to action for interested individuals to reach the next step in the clinical trial enrollment process.

All strategies considered, the number one way people obtain health-related information is by searching the web, according to CenterWatch, so it is incumbent upon clinical trial sponsors to explore this medium. Remember that social media is not an effective standalone strategy but, rather, a complementary tool for increasing study awareness. As stated by Healthcare IT News, more than 35% of Americans visit web sites such as www.clinicaltrials.gov, www.ciscrp.org and www.centerwatch.com first when accessing Facebook health resources. The U.S. federal government is seen as a credible shepherd of information.[5]

According to SAS, an expert in business analytical software, 11% of time spent on the Internet is related to social media.[6] A recent study conducted by the Pew Internet & American Life Project verified that social media is a great way to reach out to e-patients. For patients with chronic disease:

- 37% confirmed they have read someone else's notes or understanding about health-related issues via a web site, blog or online news group
- 25% have searched for reviews of hospitals and other facilities online
- 22% have signed up to receive updates on media and health-related issues
- 13% have attended a podcast about health-related topics
- 57% of e-patients living with chronic disease have done at least one of the above activities.

"Social media has the potential to connect hundreds of thousands of interested participants to clinical trials immediately," said Stanton Kawer, CEO of Blue Chip Marketing Worldwide.

While some pharmaceutical companies have not yet embraced social media, others, like Pfizer and Novartis, use this medium to unite patients and clinical trial researchers. Social media has several advantages in patient recruitment. Implementing a social media campaign provides an extra layer of contact with potential participants, but the most important part is engagement. "Social media is an excellent avenue for improving clinical trials awareness, which remains a significant barrier to recruitment," said Rahlyn Gossen of Rebar Interactive. "But harnessing the full potential of social media requires a commitment to sustained conversations with patients, as well as a departure from the "launch and leave" message broadcasting of traditional recruitment campaigns.

Other, more traditional recruitment tactics such as television and radio are costly. For example, one week of 30-second TV advertising in Chicago may cost about $15,000. Social media communities are booming and, as in the rule of supply and demand, this is a cost-effective medium.

In a recent rheumatoid arthritis study, Facebook was one of several online initiatives used to drive traffic to a study web site. Online traffic and referrals from web sites, such as Facebook and YouTube, accounted for 10% of overall study enrollment. The study enrolled two months early, because of increased study exposure to potential patients, caregivers and referring physicians. The ads appeared to individuals who indicated they were interested in seeing ads related to healthcare through the profile settings. Geo-targeting was deployed to select regions across the U.S. so only people within those regions could see the banner and print ads.

According to the April 2009 issue of *The CenterWatch Monthly*, Facebook had an overwhelming 308 groups dedicated to clinical trials. Some of these were related to specific CROs, SMOs or drug companies, but most seemed to have been developed by individuals with a particular interest in clinical trials. A June 2011 search on Facebook revealed more than 1,000 pages and groups related to clinical trials, pharmaceutical and biotech companies and individual study sites.

Does a Social Medium Work in the Clinical Trial Setting?

Medicine 2.0, the new generation of medicine, as it is referred to by the National Institutes of Health, promotes online collaboration among patients through social networking platforms. Online patient communities, such as everydayhealth.com and patientslikeme.com, encourage individuals to join communities, both mainline and disease-specific.

A Dallas, Texas, mother of a 4-year-old girl recently diagnosed with autism, Jesse, whose name has been changed for publication, said she has become involved with social media communities related to autism.

Jesse said her involvement with an online community empowered her to share her story and be strong for her family, while providing other people with information. Jesse had joined patientslikeme.com, and within six months had become an active participant in the online discussions about autism. "It has provided me a place to go when things seem out of control," she said. "It was time to tell my story and connect with others dealing with the same thing."

Another example is the Heart Truth Campaign®, sponsored by the National Heart, Lung and Blood Institute. This campaign was launched in 2009, when Facebook and Twitter hardly existed, as a small case study to test the results with social media. It was overwhelming. The Facebook page that was built in 2008 had a few individuals following the page. Once the medium expanded to Twitter, Flickr and was also supported by banner advertising and a custom web page, Facebook fans grew by 81% in one year to over 400. According to the NIH, this campaign exceeded expectations for this program. Similarly, in clinical trials giving supporters a way to show their involvement may create a greater sense of community and potentially lead to higher patient enrollment than expected.[7]

Patient education leads to empowerment, which encourages engagement, which generates interest in advancing medical science. With the overwhelming responses to technology, there is no better medium with which to educate the world on health-related topics than the internet.

Type 1 Diabetes Market Research—Patient Use of Social Media

In a recent market research survey by DAC Patient Recruitment Services of Type 1 diabetes patients and members of the First Baptist Church in Dallas, Texas, 62% of 25 respondents learned about clinical trial opportunities through the internet. Of those, 33% are currently in a clinical trial and actively seek additional information online.

In addition to learning about the study online, they also noted the web site included other information on participating in clinical trials that they found helpful in making the decision to participate. Eighty-two percent of patients confirmed they had previously requested information from their physicians about helpful web sites. This reiterates the point that people want to be educated and seek their own disease solutions, including clinical trial opportunities.

Seventy-two percent of respondents stated they access their social media pages at least once a day to check for updates. Over 60% said they are interested in health and medical-related information.

Controlling the Conversation

A common topic of conversation among pharmaceutical and biotechnology companies has been how to control the conversation if using social media. There are certain settings within some platforms that allow this feature to be de-activated.

As previously noted, bad news travels faster than good news. Bad news can affect a study and a sponsor, and shed a negative light on upcoming treatments for rare diseases. On the other hand, good news can help promote the study and the sponsor. You cannot control other people's actions, so we have to learn to manage both the negative and positive when exploring social media. Some risks may be internal and will need to be managed closely and consistently to follow Good Clinical Practice guidelines and stay within HIPAA privacy rules.

Social media platforms open up organizations to public criticism about a drug or even about something that happened at an affiliated site. This can have a positive outcome, if the blog is managed appropriately. If a patient says something negative, sponsors have an opportunity to redirect the conversation, counter inaccuracies and even change the complainant's outlook.

Ethics Committee/Review Board Guidelines

In late 2009, the FDA convened public hearings to collect information for crafting guidelines governing social media in the life sciences industry. Though 2010 and 2011 did not yield formal guidance as originally anticipated, the FDA made references within its Strategies Priorities document released in September 2010 stating social media was not a priority. In December 2011, the FDA released its first draft document on social media guidance. Although the topic is being addressed, no specific outcomes can be obtained by reviewing this information. The guidance agenda has not been published, but it seems highly unlikely additional changes will take place related to the use of social media as a whole. It could be years before the FDA takes a stand on trial recruitment via social networking. Currently, there are no regulations excluding social media as a clinical trial recruitment tool. It is, therefore, important that research professionals discuss this option with the Institutional Review Board (IRB) prior to study launch.

According to an article in CenterWatch's *CWWeekly* on March 28, 2011, 21 C.F.R. § 50.25 in Section 801 of the FDA Amendments Act of 2007 (FDAAA) requires sponsors to notify participating patients that the study will be posted online on clinicaltrials.gov. The rule became effective March 7, 2011, with full compliance required by March 7, 2012. Trials that started before March 7, 2012, will not be required to re-consent patients or include the language in the ICF. It is likely the industry will see these types of rules in the future related to specific aspects of social media.[8]

When discussing social media options with your regulatory advisement board, remember that each IRB or Ethics Committee (EC) will have its own set of policies related to this topic. According to the FDA Information Sheet *Recruiting Study Subjects*, there are guidelines to follow to ensure your social media site is in line with other recruitment initiatives that may be implemented for a specific protocol. Some guidelines to consider: Avoid any statements that may be coercive and ensure that the advertisement/web page does not promise a cure.

Any advertising for which the target audience includes prospective patients will require review by the IRB/EC prior to launch. Direct advertising can cover many media, including search engines, web sites, Facebook, LinkedIn and blogs. Advertising can include display ads, rich media ads (TV, Radio), banner ads, social network pages, blogs, tweets and text messages.

The M.D. Anderson Cancer Center recommends submitting all social media content related to the page you are preparing to launch. It is acceptable to submit multiple tweets, standard responses or any other versions you may have to support the site for the duration of the implementation timeline. By doing this, you can extend the submission process and life of the Facebook or Twitter page. This prevents having to go back to the IRB with updates.

Within the clinical trial industry, countries closely regulate social media to recruit trial participants, but this is changing every day. It is unlikely that countries will follow the same approach when it comes to using social media to market clinical trials. The regulations are meant to support each country differently. Interestingly enough, internal subject protection requirements and guidelines at the sponsor level are generally more restrictive than those of the external regulatory groups.

Global Use

The internet is a widely accepted source for recruiting patients into clinical trials, especially in the U.S. and Canada. It is also gaining popularity in Europe, Asia Pacific and Latin America. In March 2010, The Nielsen Company evaluated 10 countries to determine global web user access of social media sites. The results were incredible, to say the least. In February 2010, global web users across 10 countries spent approximately 5.5 hours a month on social media platforms, an increase from three hours from one year earlier.

Figure 2: Social network usage by country/Feb 2010 home and work

Country	Time per person (hh:mm:ss)
Average	5:27:33
Italy	6:27:53
Australia	6:25:21
U.S.	6:02:34
U.K.	5:50:56
Spain	4:50:49
Brazil	4:27:54
France	4:12:01
Germany	3:47:24
Switzerland*	3:26:00
Japan	2:37:07

*home only

Source: The Nielsen Company

Figure 3: Top three social networking sites, December 2011

Country	Site #1	Site #2	Site #3
Australia	Facebook	LinkedIn	Twitter
Austria	Facebook	Badoo	Twitter
Belgium	Facebook	Badoo	LinkedIn
Brazil	Facebook	Orkut	Badoo
Canada	Facebook	LinkedIn	Twitter
Denmark	Facebook	LinkedIn	Badoo
Finland	Facebook	LinkedIn	Twitter
France	Facebook	Badoo	Skyrock
Germany	Facebook	Wer-kennt-wen	StayFriends
India	Facebook	Orkut	Twitter
Italy	Facebook	Badoo	Twitter
Japan	Facebook	Mixi	Twitter
Netherlands	Facebook	Hyves	Twitter
Norway	Facebook	LinkedIn	Twitter
Portugal	Facebook	Orkut	LinkedIn
Sweden	Facebook	LinkedIn	Twitter
Russia	Odnoklassniki	V Kontakte	Facebook
Spain	Facebook	Tuenti	Badoo
United Kingdom	Facebook	Twitter	LinkedIn
United States	Facebook	Twitter	LinkedIn

Source: Google Trends for Websites/Alexa

While the U.S. holds the status of the largest social media network, users in Italy and Australia spent more than six hours a month on social media sites, making them the countries with the most time per month spent on related social platforms.[9]

The world map of social network use, converted above into table format, shows that Facebook is sweeping the globe. The original map was created by Vincenzo Cosenza, using Alexa and Google Trend data from June 2011. Of 134 countries analyzed, Facebook has almost 700 million users. Since December 2010, Facebook has also moved into Iran and Syria.[10]

The purpose of social media is to interconnect people. From a clinical trial perspective, it is a useful tool for both study sites and sponsors.

Web platforms exist that allow patients to be a part of an online community to sign up for information on clinical trials for a specific indication, such as PPD's clinicaltrials.com. On this site, patients can register for information on upcoming trials. In addition, physicians interested in becoming involved in clinical research can provide their information, which PPD uses to support study start-up efforts and recruitment for clinical trials.

These web sites use a therapeutic module to target individuals who actively seek online solutions for health-related concerns. Once individuals register, they will be notified of enrolling studies in their area that align with their profile.

Conclusion

Social media is a dynamic tool most of us use regularly to keep in touch with our friends and families or to stay connected with professional colleagues. With the preponderance of posts, blogs, tweets and topics, it is a challenge to keep up with the flow of information. It is evident that patients proactively seek health information online. It is also well documented that family members join online support groups to help them through the challenges of caregiving and supporting loved ones. Although the verdict is still incomplete on randomization results, the wave of social media use remains an important recruitment strategy for ongoing implementation and evaluation.

Author Biography

Kristy Wort has more than 14 years of progressively responsible experience directing multimillion dollar recruitment/retention projects. She has directed more than 80 research studies in numerous indications including rheumatology, endocrinology, dermatology, pulmonology, oncology and women's health. Many have been international in scope, deepening her understanding of global regulations, cultures and customs. Kristy is a proven relationship builder in the competitive healthcare market and has been involved in award- nominated projects through the Good Clinical Practices Journal (GCPJ) in 2008 and 2009. As Director of Project Support at DAC Patient Recruitment Services, Wort also functioned as a media specialist. Currently, as a Project Manager for Acurian, Kristy focuses on strategic solutions to further business goals and bring a new perspective to management practices within the clinical research industry. She holds a bachelor's degree in marketing from American Intercontinental University and maintains active membership in the Lupus Foundation of America and the American Diabetes Association.

References

1. Stelzner, Michael A. 2011 Social Media Marketing Industry Report. *How Marketers Are Using Social Media to Grow Their Businesses*, April 2011.

2. Van Grove, Jennifer. *Social Networking Usage Surges Globally (STATS).* Mashable Business. March 19, 2010

3. Clinical Trial Facts & Figures. Center for Information and Study on Clinical Research Participation, www.ciscrp.org/professional/facts_pat.html.

4. Brownstein, Catherine A., Brownstein, John S., Williams, David S. *The power of social media in medicine.* Nature Biotechnology 2009; 27 (888-890)

5. Healthcare IT News Staff. *Healthcare websites beat out social media as a health resource.* www.healthcareitnews.com/news/healthcare-websites-beat-out-social-media-health-resource.

6. Paine, Katie. Chaves, Mark. *Social Media Metrics. Listening, Understanding and Predicting the Impacts of Social Media on Your Business.* Presented at workshop on social media metrics presented at the eMetrics conference in San Jose, California, May 2010. www.nhlbi.nih.gov/educational/hearttruth/downloads/pdf/sm-study.pdf

7. Bhargava, Rhonit. *The FDA & Social Media: What to Expect In 2011.* Fresh influence in social media and word of mouth marketing. December 21, 2010.

8. Redfearn, Suz. *FDA requires sponsors to inform study volunteers that clinical trial information will be posted online.* CWWeekly, March 28, 2011. CenterWatch. Volume 15, issue 13.

9. Database online. The Nielsen Company, 2010. Updated October 2011.

10. *Cosenza, Vincenzo. World Map of Social Networks.* www.vincos-it/wp-content/uploads/2009/06/wmsn_animated_1024.gif.

CHAPTER NINE

Global Implications in the Recruitment of Minority Subjects

By Felicia Fuller

The emergence of personalized medicine adds a new dimension of complexity to patient recruitment, as clinical trial sponsors require study participants to meet more granular criteria, including ethnicity. Though the Human Genome Project completed in 2003 suggests humans are 99.9% similar on a molecular level, subtle variances in allele frequencies among racial groups lend credence to race as a research proxy.[1] Underscoring the relevance of targeted therapies are higher mortality and morbidity among subpopulations, as well as variability in how certain races metabolize medications.

The challenge for the drug development industry is to craft clinical trial recruitment programs that educate, resonate and inspire communities of color to become research volunteers in light of historically low participation in the United States. Experts say to achieve this, minority recruitment requires strategies that transcend traditional models.

According to Diana Anderson, Ph.D., president of DAC Patient Recruitment Services in Dallas, "It begins with understanding the experiences, values and motivations of these communities and applying that knowledge in developing core programs."

Simply inserting ethnic faces on mainstream materials, for example, is insufficient, Anderson continued. Sponsors must gain insights on everything from a community's perception of the medical establishment to how individuals receive and process information. For example, with regard to advertising, African Americans are less responsive to conceptual designs and abstract concepts, instead preferring literal messaging and pictures of people in everyday situations. Hispanics and Asians, on the other hand, favor messaging that affirms their close ties to family and culture.

"All of these factors are essential considerations when designing a recruitment campaign," Anderson asserted.

Clinicians who question the necessity of tailored communication for ethnic audiences need only consider current statistics. According to the FDA, minorities represent less than 15% of clinical trial participants.[2]

Figure 1: Examples of drug efficacy variations according to race[4]

Antipsychotic Agents—Asians demonstrated a lower threshold than whites for adverse events associated with these drugs

Aricept® (donepezil)—Shown to be more effective in black patients than others with Alzheimer's disease

BiDil® (isosorbide dinitrate/hydralazine hydrochloride)—First drug approved for marketing to a specific ethnic group; used in addition to routine heart medicines to treat heart failure in black patients

Crestor® (rosuvastatin)—Demonstrated cholesterol-lowering efficacy in blacks, Hispanics and South Asians; Asians require a lower dose while blacks need a higher dose

Iressa® (gefitinib)—Showed no overall survival benefit for lung cancer patients but extended survival by 66% in Asians

Coumadin® (warfarin)—Different dosing requirements noted for blacks, whites and Asians

"At 51% and rising, minorities represent the fastest-growing population in the United States, and we face serious health crises without real data that tell us how new therapies work in what will soon become the majority of people," said James H. Powell, M.D., CPI, principal investigator for Project I.M.P.A.C.T. (Increase Minority Participation and Awareness of Clinical Research)—a program of the National Medical Association that, since 1999, has been educating black doctors and patients about clinical research.

After all, Dr. Powell added, the role of ethnicity in drug response is well documented, as evidenced by differences in dosing requirements for blacks, Asians and whites taking warfarin among other marketed medications.

"We have the science to support the need for more minority participation. Now we have to perfect our methods for reaching these audiences," said Anderson who, drawing upon 20 years' experience, offered solutions to common minority recruitment barriers.

Challenges of Minority Recruitment:

- Fear and mistrust due to:
  - Lack of knowledge about clinical research
  - Historical abuses
  - Familial objections
- Low minority physician population in the United States
- Socio-economic barriers
  - Exposure

  - Finances
  - Transportation

Solutions to Minority Recruitment Challenges:

- Educate community gatekeepers (pastors, social activists, local politicians, business owners and media personalities) who might influence ethnic audiences
- Advertise in ethnic media, including newspapers, magazines and radio
- Deploy targeted community outreach initiatives
  - Empowerment conferences
  - Fraternity and sorority events
  - Minority Health Day events
  - Church and community center health fairs
- Enlist community leaders to be the "face" of the project at outreach events
- Ensure that clinical staff is diverse and reflects the population served
  - Tap in to minority physicians groups such as the National Medical Association
- Ensure subjects receive clear information on what to expect during and after a study
- Ensure messaging:
  - Reflects positive images of ethnic life
  - Features people in "real" situations, not talking heads
  - Depicts people of different skin tones and hair textures

Beyond advertising tactics, education and outreach are essential, as Dr. Philip Gorelick, director of the center for stroke research and head of the department of neurology and rehabilitation at the University of Illinois College of Medicine in Chicago, discovered. Dr. Gorelick was principal investigator of the African-American Antiplatelet Stroke Prevention Study (AAASPS), the first large-scale recurrent stroke study of African Americans. The multicenter, randomized, double-blind clinical trial was testing the efficacy of ticlopidine (500 mg/day) with aspirin (650 mg/day) in preventing recurrent stroke, vascular death and myocardial infarction.

Before launching the trial, Dr. Gorelick and his colleagues developed an intricate recruitment strategy that included cultural sensitivity training for site staff and community buy-in initiatives, as well as demographic and psychographic analyses to identify and overcome barriers to trial participation.

From these efforts emerged what AAASPS researchers identified as the "recruitment triangle," early predictors of patients' likelihood to participate in and remain compliant with clinical research. Sides of the triangle included the patient, key family members and friends and the primary medical doctor and other medical personnel.[3]

"By maintaining the integrity of the recruitment triangle, refusal and premature voluntary withdrawal may be minimized," Dr. Gorelick and his colleagues wrote in an interim report published in the *Journal of the National Medical Association*. "Social support, education about the research and development of trust can sever the barriers and serve as the glue of the recruitment triangle."

AAASPS investigators at 62 sites enrolled 1,809 African-American subjects over the course of the trial, which began in 1995 and ended in 2001 when interim analysis revealed lack of efficacy. Despite its end, few studies today can compare to the precedent set by the AAASPS.

A History of Underrepresentation

For years researchers have debated why fewer ethnic minorities participate in clinical trials compared to the white population. Some cite past injustices, such as the now-infamous Tuskegee experiment, for perceived distrust of the medical establishment by African Americans in particular. In this U.S.-sponsored research to examine the natural progression of syphilis, 600 black sharecroppers from Alabama—399 who already had syphilis and 201 without the disease—were told they had "bad blood" and, enticed with the promise of free medical care, enrolled in the study and were allowed to go untreated from 1932 to 1972. Many of the men died, while others unwittingly passed the disease to their wives, many of whom gave birth to babies with congenital syphilis.

"We can't forget Tuskegee, because it is part of the African-American experience and its negative impact shaped the outlook of a generation," said Mona Fouad, M.D., M.P.H., professor and director of the Division of Preventive Medicine at the University of Alabama in Birmingham. As a result, she added, the prospect of participating in clinical research aimed at ethnic communities raises suspicion and fear, with many questioning the motivation.

Dr. Jean G. Ford, director of the Johns Hopkins Center to Reduce Cancer Disparities, concurred, saying, "The Tuskegee incident is a salient historical event that crystalized people's perceptions that they've been treated unfairly. It's significant because it symbolizes something consistent with cultural orientation based on a history of oppression."

Yet such injustices in the name of science are not limited to U.S. borders. From 1946 to 1948, the U.S. funded clinical research in South America in which prostitutes were used to infect 700 Guatemalan prisoners and mental patients with syphilis, purportedly to test the effectiveness of penicillin to treat the disease.

In response to revelations about the Guatemalan tragedy, President Barack Obama signed an Executive Order in November 2009 creating the Presidential Commission for the Study of Bioethical Issues—a body of international experts commissioned to review and report on the most effective methods to ensure all human medical research conducted around the globe meets rigorous ethical standards. The commission is headed by Dr. Amy Gutmann, a scholar on ethics and public policy who currently serves as president of the University of Pennsylvania.

U.S. Secretary of State Hillary Clinton and Health and Human Services Secretary Kathleen Sebelius issued an apology to the Guatemalan government in October 2010 for the U.S. Public Health Service Sexually Transmitted Disease Inoculation Study, calling it "unethical" and "appalling."

"Things are changing in some ways and it is possible that in subsequent generations, Tuskegee [and other events like it] will cease to have impact," Dr. Ford said.

While medical atrocities fuel suspicion and fear among some individuals, recent data suggest minority involvement in clinical research may be more closely linked to access than attitudes.

The same dynamic applies globally. Some trial leaders supply all investigational product and comparators to ROW countries, which can be logistically more challenging. It is indicative of the healthcare issue or level of standard of care. In some ROW countries the comparators are beyond reach in the general population (and more so in ethnic populations) due to expense.

According to researchers at the National Institutes of Health (NIH) and Yale School of Medicine, minorities in the U.S. participate in clinical trials at the same rate as whites when they meet study criteria and are informed about the opportunity to enroll.[5]

"The real problems are inadequate culturally appropriate information and ineffective effort—both of which perpetuate health disparities along racial lines in this country," Dr. Powell said. "From institutional review boards to informed consent, many advances have been made to correct the issues that were so blatant during the Tuskegee incident. We have to educate people in a culturally appropriate manner so they understand the value of clinical trials and their protections in the process."

Dr. Fouad agreed, stating, "We can't be sure doctors are offering trial opportunities to everyone. By educating communities concerning clinical research, we empower patients so they can be their own advocates and ask doctors about their trial eligibility."

The Role of Doctors

Fundamental to the push to improve ethnic participation is soliciting the support of minority physicians who, according to population studies, have profound influence on their patients' health choices. However, racial inequities in research mirror low minority physician representation nationwide.

For context, black doctors comprise less than 4% of U.S. physicians, according to recent data from the Association of American Medical Colleges.[6] Dr. Powell estimates that of approximately 30,000 black U.S. physicians, less than 1% conducts clinical trials.

"Even though we are 47 years removed from the Civil Rights Act, medicine is largely still segregated in the United States," said Dr. Ford. "Investigators, who are mainly funded by the National Institutes of Health, are not generally people of color and do not understand how to reach people in communities where they have no history. They simply are not congruent with the culture. Physicians of color bring more clarity to the strategies and help overcome incorrect assumptions about the community being targeted for research."

Dr. Powell theorizes that minority doctors, many of whom work in underserved communities, are interested in becoming principal investigators but are stymied by lack of time and resources.

A survey of 1,400 doctors conducted by the Tufts Center for the Study of Drug Development at Tufts University found that 16.9% of white physicians participated as principal investigators in clinical trials compared to 14% of black physicians. The results, published in the 2006 *Tufts CSDD Impact Report*, also found that:[7]

- More than half of black (51%) and Hispanic (57%) physicians consider a physician's race an important factor in influencing minority patient participation in clinical research, compared to white physicians (9%)
- Minority physicians are less likely to refer their patients into clinical studies than white physicians (38% vs. 47%, respectively).
- Minority physicians perceive barriers to their participation as investigators at similar levels to their white counterparts. These barriers include time constraints, personnel and infrastructure needs.

Regardless of ethnic persuasion, Dr. Fouad said doctors must equitably inform eligible patients about clinical trial opportunities.

To that end, the National Cancer Institute's Minority-Based Community Clinical Oncology Program requires 40% minority representation among cancer patients enrolled in its research. In 2003, the MB-CCOPs accounted for less than 20% of the CCOP network but enrolled half the minority participants. Its strategy includes partnering with community clinics and permitting research participants to see their family physicians rather than having to travel to study sites for tests and procedures. This helps combat barriers associated with travel, site accessibility and doctor rapport.

"MB-CCOPs are successful because of minority doctor involvement," Dr. Ford explained.

Beyond U.S. Borders

The quest for diversity has prompted many biopharmaceutical companies to conduct clinical trials in populous, treatment-naïve regions outside North America, including India, Africa, Asia and South America. For example, while Hispanics are the largest ethnic group in America, they are underrepresented in U.S. research. In response, the FDA advocates research expansion to Latin American countries such as Brazil, Argentina and Mexico.

Brazil

Most notably, Brazil's strength as a clinical research center lies in its ethnically diverse population of 203 million people. Among them, 53.7% are white, 38.5% are mulatto (or mixed-race), 6.2% are black, 9% identify as "other" (i.e., Japanese, Arab, Amerindian), and 7% are unspecified. Isolated indigenous tribes comprise less than 1% of the population. With illiteracy rates hovering near 10%, largely along ethnic lines, trial sponsors must take calculated steps to protect patients' rights and facilitate their understanding of the research process.

To date, Brazil's efforts in the research realm have proven successful. The country's pharmaceutical market index boasts a 14.5% compound annual growth rate forecast through 2014. Additionally, Brazil is home to South America's first academic research organization, the Brazilian Clinical Research Institute (BCRI), located on the Federal University campus in San Paulo.

In general, Latin America offers high recruitment rates, a compliant retention environment due to close physician-patient relationships, strong physician knowledge of and adherence to ICH-GCP guidelines and consistency with Western medicine standards. Conducting successful trials in the region requires a local presence that understands approval guidelines and standards. Regulatory review can be lengthy and, in contrast to North America, unexpected protocol concerns and occasional difficulties in resolving queries surface more frequently.

India

India has a large, genetically diverse, treatment-naïve patient population experiencing an emergence of common Western diseases. As in many ROW societies, physicians play a pivotal, almost paternalistic, role in the lives of their patients and greatly influence their healthcare decisions. Another factor clinical trial leaders have noted is the need for ongoing investigator training. Because they lack knowledge of regulations, ethics, GCP and skills for clinical trial management, the trial quality is inconsistent. Inadequate permanent research staff and poor infrastructure for drug/sample storage are additional considerations. With 14 official languages, accurate translation of patient-facing documents also presents a formidable challenge.

South Africa

South Africa provides an ethnically diverse population for a broader spectrum of clinical trial data. According to recent census figures, the racial breakdown includes black African, 79%; white, 9.6%; mixed race (black African and European), 8.9%; and Indian/Asian, 2.5%. Other regional advantages are English-speaking medical professionals, several established research sites and a large treatment-naïve population with varied prevalence of infectious diseases—a mix of first- and third-world diseases. Though public awareness about clinical trials is strong, there are difficulties obtaining government consent to initiate placebo studies in indications for which there is an approved treatment.

Malaysia

Malaysia is a source of multi-ethnic subjects representing two larger Asian markets—India and China. Educational programs have been instituted and promoted in the country, which have enhanced the knowledge of investigators conducting clinical trials. In addition, because English is widely spoken in Malaysia, business may be executed more efficiently.

Despite the known advantages of conducting clinical trials in ROW countries, many challenges remain. These include lack of experienced investigators, long regulatory cycle times, high monitoring cost, different standard of care doses for comparators, issues with healthcare delivery systems, lack of manpower or specialists, poor outreach campaigns, inadequate resources, low educational levels and cultural and religious barriers.

To overcome these global hurdles, translation and localization expertise must be employed. Ethical practices must be improved so international standards are maintained. Ethnically and culturally sensitive patient recruitment campaigns must be deployed. Finally, regulatory awareness must be heightened so trial sponsors can proceed with greater clarity and experience greater success. If there is adequate and open communication with healthcare providers, project team members and recruitment teams/vendors about cultural barriers, recruitment can be successful. Partnering with community-based organizations during the planning and development phase of a clinical project is also a key determinant of recruitment outcomes.

Strategies for targeting diverse populations globally include enlistment of investigators from the targeted ethnic group, collaboration with community organizations, use of culturally competent advertisement and acculturation of clinical trial staff. At one large global company, medical teams partner with investigators in ROW countries to ascertain their clinical research expertise. Additionally, ROW key opinion leaders (KOLs) are involved in the feasibility process for upcoming protocols "to tap their input and interest."

Mobilizing Forces

On Aug. 3, 2010, the National Medical Association convened its annual meeting and scientific assembly in Orlando, Fla. The event theme, *Race Matters: Patients, Doctors and Clinical Trials*, focused on strategies for increasing minority representation among research subjects and trial investigators. From that meeting, Dr. James H. Powell and his team at Project I.M.P.A.C.T. announced plans to develop a survey focused on minority research participation. Discussions continued during the association's 2011 annual meeting in Washington, D.C., under the banner, *Health Equity: Lead, Reform, Deliver.* Yolanda Fleming, project director at I.M.P.A.C.T., said program officials are seeking logistical support and funding to execute survey plans.

Meanwhile, progress is being made in the Enhancing Minority Participation in Clinical Trials (EMPaCT) program announced by the University of Minnesota Medical School in 2010, funded with a $3.8 million grant from the National Institutes of Health's National Center on Minority Health and Health Disparities (NCMHD). EMPaCT aims to address the barriers and biases that limit minority participation and access to clinical trials via research conducted by academic institutions in five regions: Johns Hopkins University (east), University of Alabama at Birmingham (southeast), University of Minnesota (midwest), University of Texas M.D. Anderson Cancer Center (south) and University of California, Davis (west).

EMPaCT's lead investigator is Dr. Selwyn M. Vickers, the University of Minnesota's associate director of translational research, and Jay Phillips, professor and chairman in the Department of Surgery. Dr. Vickers is nationally renown in pancreatic cancer research, more specifically, gene therapy for treating pancreatobiliary tumors and the role of growth factors and receptors in pancreatic cancer. Dr. Mona Fouad of the University of Alabama and Dr. Jean Ford of Johns Hopkins University are among six investigators supporting Dr. Vickers in the EMPaCT program from their academic institutions.

"We're trying to go beyond the barriers that have been reported in the literature, and community barriers like lack of trust and accessibility," Dr. Fouad said. "We are developing networks of cancer centers in every region of the country and working through them to understand systemic challenges concerning minority recruitment within the cancer centers themselves. Once we know more we can find models that can work within the system."

Efforts began with qualitative data mined from interviews with cancer center directors, research nurses and administrators. Research results revealed during the EMPaCT national meeting on July 29, 2011, in Bethesda, Maryland, underscored the following chief areas of concern:

1. **Lack of diversity training among research staff**
   Cancer center staff, including research nurses and investigators, were asked, "Have you been trained, educated or become aware of how to combat minority enrollment issues in clinical trials?" Most said they receive no guidance on how to enhance minority participation. "There has to be some kind of educational component before recruitment for

the trial begins," said Dr. Fouad. "I recommend web-based programs over in-person training to accommodate physicians' busy schedules and ensure strong participation."

2. **Inadequate retention strategies**
   Dr. Fouad said physicians and nurses rightfully focus on regulatory requirements and the rudiments of research, but they often neglect to proactively craft strategies to establish patient support systems and counter compliance issues. Patient turnover can yield inadequate data to accurately analyze study findings.

Maintaining a competitive edge requires a detailed participant retention plan, which evolves from analyses of similar studies and market research focused on patients who meet study criteria. Developing a process to identify and screen potential participants who are likely to be non-compliant or who may drop out also serves to augment efforts.

"Participating in a clinical trial carries a lot of responsibility," Dr. Fouad said. "Patients have to visit the research center frequently, sometimes weekly, and they have to undergo a battery of examinations and tests. If they don't have reliable transportation, they can't follow trial requirements. Some don't have jobs that will permit them to take off. Insurance coverage may be limited and may not pay for clinical trial expenses. I know from experience that patients are embarrassed to talk about such things—to say, 'I don't have a car. I don't have money to pay for gas to get here.' We should ask about these things and have a plan for addressing them."

Discerning financial and family challenges among some ethnic groups may be difficult due to cultural norms placing particular emphasis on personal pride or privacy. Therefore, Dr. Fouad suggested, clinicians must be culturally astute and communication savvy.

To maintain interest and reinforce compliance among trial participants at the University of Alabama, she and her team have developed what they term a "navigation model." First, the team conducts educational events at clinics in minority communities to inform physicians and patients about clinical trial opportunities. A patient who expresses an interest in participation, and who qualifies on pre-screening, is paired with a member of the research team known as the navigator. During informed consent, the navigator is present to explain the IC document in layman's language and answer any questions from the patient and his or her family. The navigator also identifies and addresses possible retention barriers, acts as liaison between the patient and the insurance company if necessary and links the patient with support groups for individuals with the same disease indication.

So far, the navigation model has proven successful—so much so that the University of Alabama submitted a grant proposal in June 2011 suggesting similar models as a continuation of EMPaCT.

"We must seek to understand the community, lifestyle, behaviors and cultural values of minority patients, including those in urban, suburban and rural environments," said Dr. Fouad. "Researchers can't take anything for granted."

Anderson lauded the efforts of EMPaCT and similar programs, saying, "If our messages don't reach the right audiences, they don't participate. If they don't participate, we're left with inadequate data. With inadequate data, our health system is at risk. Inadequate data is simply not an option."

Author Biographies

Felicia Fuller is Publications Manager for DAC Patient Recruitment Services, an Imperial company, leading the editorial development of all client and corporate promotional collateral, including print, broadcast and online content targeted to clinical and lay audiences. She is a published writer with 19 years of experience in multiple industries, having worked as a newspaper reporter, magazine editor and corporate publications strategist. Felicia won a 2011 Hermes Award for the article, "A Question of Color: Overcoming Barriers to Minority Research Participation."

Contributing writer Karen Brooks is currently pursuing her doctorate in International Health Practitioner from TUI University. Previously, she was Senior Director of Project Delivery at PRA International, focusing on the client relationship and management of key preferred provider relationships, and Director of Clinical Projects at sanofi. Karen serves as a board member for Trinity Research Consultants, a specialty SMO focused on novice minority investigators.

References

1. Satel, Sally. *Race and Medicine Can Mix Without Prejudice: How the Story of BiDil Illuminates the Future of Medicine*. Medical Progress Today. December 10, 2004. Available at: www.medicalprogresstoday.com/spotlight/spotlight_indarchive.php?id=449. Accessed June 2011.

2. U.S. Food and Drug Administration.

3. Gorelick, Philip; Harris, Yvonne; Burnett, Barbara; Bonecutter, Faith J. *The Recruitment Triangle: Reasons Why African Americans Enroll, Refuse to Enroll, or Voluntarily Withdraw from a Clinical Study*. Journal of the National Medical Association, Vol. 90, No. 3; 141-145.

4. Osagie K. Obasogie, *Playing the Gene Card: A Report on Race and Human Biotechnology*. Oakland: Center for Genetics and Society, 2009. Available at: www.geneticsandsociety.org/downloads/complete_PTGC.pdf. Accessed June 20, 2011.

5. *Minority Participation in Health Research—Facts and Fiction*. PLoS Med 3(2). December 6, 2005.

6. Association of American Medical Colleges.
7. Tufts CSDD Impact Report, 2006.
8. The World Fact Book. U.S. Central Intelligence Agency. Available online at www.cia.gov/library/publications/the-world-factbook. Accessed July 19, 2011.

CHAPTER TEN

The Sponsor Perspective: Developing Continuity of Recruitment Processes Across Therapeutic Indications

By Joe Kim

The Earth is not Global

How could something made from the "best stuff on earth" not be universally enjoyed? In the early 1970s, a small American company called Snapple was born and grew steadily over the following decades, using the catchy slogan, "Made from the Best Stuff on Earth" and quirky, off-beat marketing to gain popularity in a market in which the next best thing was a metallic, cloying version of brewed tea in a can.

Snapple reached the pinnacle of popular culture in 1993 when it landed a reference on the hit U.S. television sitcom, *Seinfeld*. Although the reference was less than unabashedly promotional—something along the lines of it's "too fruity,"—Snapple had, by all other accounts, arrived.

Shortly after its appearance on *Seinfeld*, Snapple was acquired by the Quaker Oats Company with the promise of global expansion. Setting its sites on Japan—at the time and still today, one of the leading soft drink markets in the world—Quaker took Snapple into the Asian market with the marketing strategy of simply leveraging its American-ness.

What happened next has been discussed in countless business articles and books, so I will not belabor the point. Suffice it to say the Japanese Snapple strategy, or lack thereof, is a perfect example of what not to do in global marketing. Basically, what made Snapple successful in the United States is what made it fail in Japan.

The Japanese reaction to Snapple ultimately was negative. The heavy glass bottles didn't translate in the portable vending machine culture. The quantity was too great, the flavor was overpowering and, most of all, the Japanese did not like cloudy tea. Whereas in the U.S., the cloudiness was attributed to natural elements (e.g., pulp), the Japanese found it off-putting. Unable to react quickly to consumer feedback, we can only imagine the level of investment Snapple made before it was too late. In the mid 1990s the Internet was little more than a system to house an unlimited number of electronic billboards. There was no way to actively "listen" to consumers en masse. Had there been the sophisticated functionality that exists today, Snapple may have been able to get ahead of these issues and course correct without having to limp out of Japan.

Fast forward to the present and readily pick up real customer feedback on Snapple's current efforts, as well as find evidence the company has learned its lesson. Below is a quote from the Japanese section of the online food blog, Biggestmenu.com.

> "Now I'm not sure whether or not Snapple has milk tea in the U.S., but for me, it was a first. My brother bought this at a vending machine in Japan, and it was surprisingly tasty!"
>
> —*Biggestmenu.com*

All of the issues that plagued the mid-'90s version of Snapple are gone—smaller size, aluminum can and, now clearly emblazoned on the label, the terms "healthy and **clear**." But the quote shows that Snapple still has to overcome doubts and fears about its products. Whether this can be attributed to its initial failure is tough to know.

So what does iced tea have to do with patient recruitment? Absolutely nothing.

International marketing, however, has everything to do with patient recruitment. Both take discipline, time and a reverence for the customer, or, in this case, patient-centric principles. Put another way, successful patient recruitment starts by working from a patient-centric perspective and allowing time to take a disciplined approach to first understand the patient. Only with this approach can industry professionals devise effective strategies and tactics to raise awareness and instill a call-to-action in a way that is reproducible across geographies and therapeutic areas.

We are not in the Business of Science

The initial reactions to this philosophy and approach are usually characterized by phrases like "there's no time," "our scientific advisory board understands this patient population like no one else" or "this isn't marketing." While it may be true that there is not a great deal of time available (in fact, there is never a great deal of time), there is certainly always time to understand customers, especially when the clinical trials industry engages them so intimately and so far in advance of commercialization. Fast food corporations do a fantastic job engaging and understanding customers during the research and development process. Given that the biopharmaceutical industry works to help deliver medicines that improve people's lives, does the industry not owe it to patients to exceed the efforts of those who may contribute to the exact problems science tries to solve? The biopharmaceutical industry is one characterized by constant innovation insofar as the core function is to discover, develop and commercialize new therapies. Other industries that are defined by this kind of innovation—for example, the best Silicon Valley technology firms—espouse a very intimate feedback loop with their customer base and have built it into the development process. There must be time for this.

Another commonly heard comment against the patient-centric recruitment model is usually associated with the idea that scientists best know the patient population and so there may be no need to do further work in this area. The real issue here is that there is confusion among the following elements: knowledge of the disease, the compound and the patient. It may be true that key opinion leaders understand the disease like no one else. It certainly is true that the sponsor's scientists best understand the pharmacokinetics and pharmacodynamics of the investigational drug. However, only the patients themselves truly understand their own behaviors and issues as they relate to their conditions on a daily basis. And without a halfway decent characterization gathered from data provided by patients, recruitment strategies will remain suboptimal as they will suffer from diverging viewpoints and weak foundations.

The most often used rebuttal, which also happens to be the most invalid, is when clinical teams deny their roles as marketers. The best organizations realize that everyone is in sales and marketing. Can you imagine if the FDA required all new formulations of soft drinks to be tested on humans prior to launch, to ensure they were tasty and accessible by all? Does anyone think for one moment that a soft drink firm would stack a research team for this purpose with mere chemists, supply chain professionals and distribution gurus alone? There is no doubt marketers would hold a prominent role on these research teams to better understand the customer, especially during the research phase. I am not suggesting we recruit marketing professionals to help clinical research teams conduct studies. But because the industry has prospered in the past with a less-than-robust patient-centric approach during development does not mean it should continue to do so. Biopharmaceutical industry professionals are not in the business of science. They are in the science business. And all good businesses place the customer at the center.

Chances are Someone isn't Sharing

The foundation of a patient-centric recruitment model comprises two main elements: 1) a patient portrait and 2) a patient pathway. The patient portrait is simply a description of the patient's major influences, drivers, issues, concerns, outlets, hopes, fears, etc. There are numerous ways to both gather this data and frame it for consumption, but traditional methods usually call for a mix of in-depth interviews, focus groups and surveys. Bolstering or informing this research is any number of secondary data sets relevant to demographic characteristics, other consumer behaviors and technological penetration, to name a few. However, given the rich content appearing in social media forums, discussion boards and health activist blogs, additional techniques of "listening" could be leveraged to gather a complete picture up front as well as to track evolving trends and reactions. While it is virtually impossible to manually scour the Internet for this information, there are various providers that leverage technology to gather this data and parse it out with relative ease.

The framework to summarize and present a patient portrait is fairly loose and certainly flexible enough to suit the needs of an organization. Whatever the final format, it is critical to ensure the final analysis is distilled into clear characterizations, so actionable recommendations to either amplify elements of the patient portrait or mitigate the impact of challenges can be properly aligned and clearly articulated. Identification of root causes also may be critical to establish a convincing rationale for action. For example, it is commonly understood that patients with ulcerative colitis may feel reluctant to stray far from their geographic comfort zone. While this is an important detail, the root cause, i.e., the ability to mitigate the risk of gastrointestinal "accidents," is more critical to the patient portrait than the idea of the "restricted travel range" alone. Cultural differences may affect the severity or alter the final behavior, so these need to be taken into account as well.

If time and resources are scare, one could effectively create a limited recruitment support strategy based on the patient portrait alone. These recommendations could manifest as deceivingly simple solutions or rather obvious sophisticated tactics. For example, another common understanding is that newly diagnosed HIV patients often undergo a transformational, personal experience upon knowledge of their diagnosis, much akin to a religious conversion. Turning a finding like this into actionable recommendations can be tricky. And leveraging this data into concrete executions can be as simple as influencing the phrasing of the tagline on a poster or acting as the impetus to develop a complex physician and family relationship guide for the newly diagnosed. Of course, these decisions are not straightforward, and choosing which recommendation to implement is mainly a function of the talent of the recruitment strategist, past experience, timing and, of course, a bit of luck.

The patient pathway (a.k.a. "patient journey" or "patient healthcare utilization model") is essentially a step-by-step understanding of how a patient may move among various touch points before coming to a final diagnosis. Depending on the indication, these touch points may include personal influencers, over-the-counter remedies, medical or paramedical resources and interventions of a holistic or alternative nature. Once diagnosed, the patient pathway should also articulate the various treatment pathways and disease management activities taken by the patient. While this should be focused on the standard of care, it should also give weight to patient behaviors. For example, if it is well known that patients become non-compliant with a chronic medication for a certain indication, this should be called out. Or perhaps patients may severely restrict social activity as a result of disease symptoms, so this would need to be stated. Additionally, where there may be a selection of alternatives, it is important that the pathway attempts to articulate the distribution between or among the alternatives (e.g., 50/50; 70/30; 10/30/60). This distribution helps to illuminate the relative sizes of the differing patient segments and will, therefore, inform the decision to actively design segment-specific strategies to reach these patients or whether to pursue at all.

Due to the inevitable loops and branching that occur during a patient's journey, the ideal framework to depict a patient pathway may take the form of a process map or flow chart. Unfortunately, well-established patient pathway archetypes do not seem to exist in the public domain, so there are no standard templates one could leverage. To make matters worse, the time required to develop one can be challenging given the myriad inputs and opinions required to deliver a rigorous enough model for the team to accept. Finally, clinical researchers are not accustomed to this kind of formal activity, both operationally and intellectually. Researchers understand data tables, pharmacokinetic curves and box and whisker plots. Market segmentation is not part of their common vernacular. But remember, biopharmaceutical organizations are commercial in nature. The good news is that unless one works for an early-phase start-up biotech that is not planning to commercialize a compound in-house, most companies will have an entire team dedicated to this kind of research. More often than not, patient portraits and pathways are being formulated on a daily basis. They just haven't been shared with the research teams.

However, in this day and age it would be foolish to engage in a proof-of-concept or late-stage suite of trials without at least having some baseline understanding of the market and the customers—patients, providers and payers. And while some business rules may dictate this research take place upon achieving proof-of-concept, for a cost equivalent to enrolling several extra patients as per the patient grant, teams could develop and leverage a more robust understanding of the patient that would yield quicker enrollment cycle times. And if proof-of-concept is achieved, commercial teams can use this market research as a springboard to deeper knowledge more quickly than if they had not done initial research.

Planning is Everything, Plans are Nothing

There are many instances in life when the nature of how things are done is just as important as the end result. Take a typical Western legal system. Indeed, all have their faults. They are often slow, bloated and prone to some level of corruption. However, the concept of due process always holds sway over pure speed and accuracy. While the accused may be quite obviously guilty of a crime because of clear forensic evidence, it is still important that stakeholders respect due process. Arguably, the process is sometimes more important than the end results. In short, this is the opposite of an "ends justify the means" philosophy. Patient recruitment strategy development is no different.

When patient recruitment professionals aim to develop strategies across indications, and across cultures and regions, this concept of showing reverence for the process is important. Yes, it requires discipline and patience, but it should pay dividends in the long run, both when things go well and when they do not go as planned.

When a recruitment strategy derails, initial instincts may drive stakeholders to blame the tactics themselves as well as the decisions to use those tactics. And if there are no standard planning tools to reference, team members, vendors and customers often end up in a finger-pointing standoff, with efforts not focused on optimizing results, but instead focused on massaging data, combing through old emails or writing memoirs with the hope of minimizing any personal blame. With no evidence of cogent thinking or conspicuous buy-in, survival mode kicks in. When that happens, individuals scramble to avoid being hanged, rather than working to hang together.

Prevention of this scenario can be improved by adhering to the recruitment strategy principles discussed above. Team members must remain aligned in a rationale that has been crystallized in a clear format, based on patient drivers as the foundation. If done well, the root causes of derailment are usually finite and limited to an imperfect characterization of the patient and the patient pathway or an imprecise estimation of projected results. Because of the numerous permutations of patient characterizations and the ever-changing landscape of healthcare and clinical research, mitigating these risks is nearly impossible. As such, gaining agreement on the assumptions that drive these elements becomes that much more critical. The more teams can be transparent in their assumptions, thinking and final endorsement, the more likely individuals will move beyond the arguably defensible mistakes, and instead spend energy on remediation when things go wrong. Because they will.

As former U.S. President Dwight D. Eisenhower said, "Planning is everything, plans are nothing."

So it's Just Like Marketing, Only not Really

Developing a strategy to recruit patients in clinical trials can appear to be eerily similar to tactics used when devising a marketing campaign for consumer goods and services. However, the unfortunate truth is that patient recruitment strategies have little time to evolve due to the relatively brief nature of clinical trial enrollment cycle times in comparison to commercial marketing campaigns. As a result, the pressures and subsequent decisions in this context are somewhat unusual and counterintuitive to the traditional marketer. And so while much of what was discussed indeed represents some core elements of a traditional marketing discipline, on the ground the finishing moves can be somewhat different.

For example, let's say an online keyword campaign is being used to reach patients seeking trial-related healthcare information on the Internet. The commercial marketer may show an instinctive desire to analyze the performance of each keyword combination and bid price to maximize the responses from the right patient segment, continuously adding or subtracting keywords and altering bids in hopes of seeking the optimum mix. While this is the right approach for a persistent consumer brand, clinical trial marketers do not have that kind of luxury and so need to go very wide and continue with seemingly "poor performing" keyword combinations. The reason is, even if a handful of patients click through, screen and ultimately randomize, the keyword combinations would have paid off. In clinical research, progress is not measured in percentage points. Every patient counts.

What is the Nature of the Game?

American football is said to be a game of inches. Restaurants, a game of pennies. The most basic distillation of variables driving the success and failure of those who may choose to play in any domain is important to understand, and clinical trial recruitment is no different. Patient recruitment is a game of patients. They drive assumptions, strategy and tactics. Enrollment rates are measured in patients, per site, per month. Each one matters and is accounted for at the integer level. Without them there is no data, no customer and no industry.

Author Biography

Joseph Kim is Clinical Operations Director at Shire, focusing on developing and implementing innovative trial optimization solutions in a heavily outsourced model. He has spent 13 years in the pharma industry utilizing a unique approach that integrates his experiences working for Sponsors, CROs and niche vendors. As a former member of Merck's Global Trial Optimization leadership team, he was a key contributor to helping the organization secure the industry's top spot in PA-LPI cycle time. He has the rare combination of experience that includes early and late-phase clinical research and a command of IT-related solutions and development models. Joseph holds a B.S. in Molecular Biology from Lehigh University and an MBA from Villanova.

CHAPTER ELEVEN

The U.S. Site Perspective on Organized Patient Recruitment Challenges and Opportunities

By Christine Pierre

So often we hear the number one reason studies are delayed in meeting their deadline is related to the slow enrollment of study subjects. Many believe sluggish efforts of North American sites to meet enrollment goals has caused sponsors to seek support from research sites throughout the rest of the world. It is estimated that between 40% and 65% of all clinical studies are being conducted outside of the United States.[1]

Cleary many lessons have been learned within the North American borders that can be applied to research sites around the globe. It would be a shame for sites and others to not share the best practices they have uncovered as successful tools to be implemented at research sites to ensure the studies we are conducting meet targeted enrollment goals and timelines.

Assessing the root cause of enrollment delays is heavily influenced by your vantage point.

From the public's perspective, while people are willing to participate to help build knowledge and find cures, they say they seldom are notified of study opportunities. And while study participation begets deep appreciation and satisfaction, many patients say new treatments are too expensive and take too long to develop.

Moving beyond laying blame on the other party, let's discover and commit to implementing best recruitment practices that can be utilized by all to have a positive impact on the recruitment results of any study.

Protocol Design

The rapid changes being implemented within clinical practice certainly make drafting a study protocol something that should not be done within a corporate vault or laboratory. Nor should its external input rely solely on the

Figure 1

Site's perspective	Sponsor's perspective	Public's perspective
Poor protocol design	Sites failing to conduct a thorough study feasibility	Seldom notified of study opportunities
Being asked to commit to a study before having a final protocol	Sites lacking a recruitment plan	Willing to participate to help build body of knowledge and find cures
Inadequate recruitment budget	Sites unable to execute a recruitment plan	New treatments are too expensive and take too long to develop
Outside recruitment firms sending potential subjects that do not fit the protocol	Sites not following up on potential subjects identified by an outside recruitment firm	Study participation begets deep appreciation and satisfaction

advice of Key Opinion Leaders (KOL). Neither of these groups has the full understanding of clinical practice "in the real world today," and some lack the first-hand experience of working with study volunteers. Critical insight would be gained by including input from clinical research professionals conducting clinical research today during the protocol design phase. To overlook the opportunity to include clinical research professionals who are taking care of patients and conducting clinical research when designing a protocol is a missed and potentially very costly mistake for the sponsor.

Beyond the clinical elements of any study protocol are the mechanics of the protocol—specifically, things that affect and or involve the study subject, such as the use of electronic diaries, the length and frequency of visits and the variety of tests and procedures requested of them. While the scientist may view these events as mere means to an end, potential subjects may view them as deal breakers in volunteering for a clinical study, and research staff may decline the study for similar reasons.

By utilizing currently involved research site professionals' input during the protocol design phase, the end results could be the opportunity to develop a more implementable protocol. While nothing will remove all obstacles intrinsic to a difficult study, the inclusion of input from those who execute studies on the front line can lead to reducing prolonged study timelines, which leads to crippling financial statements and ultimately causes excessive delays in providing new treatments to our patients.

Study Feasibility

It is estimated that approximately 60% of research sites complete one to three site questionnaires each week, and fewer than 5% spend more than one hour

Figure 2: Distribution of delays in U.S. site enrollment timelines

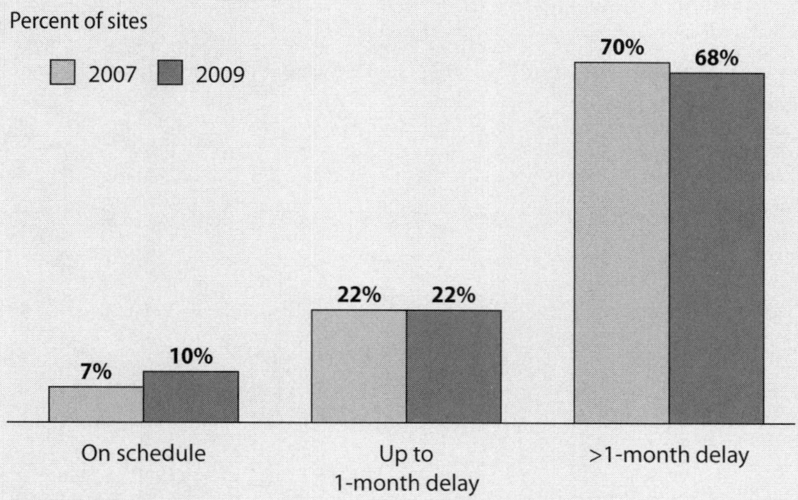

Source: CenterWatch 2009 (N=950), 2007 (N=522), Surveys of U.S. Investigative Sites

completing the form.[2] During this stage, the site is typically provided with little more than a study synopsis. However, the fundamental question the sender is asking—how many potential subjects can you enroll in a set period of time—rests squarely and heavily on everyone's shoulders. How sites arrive at the answer to that very critical question varies, from their gut reaction to past performance on similar studies and database verification.[3] Clearly, the past has highlighted that these methods leave much to be desired, given that 70% of all study subjects come from 30% of all sites[4], and almost 70% of all studies run more than a month beyond their targeted enrollment deadline.[5] (See Figure 2).

The recent evolution of the Electronic Medical Record (EMR) has single-handedly provided research sites the greatest aid not only in determining the answer to the question of how many potential subjects they can enroll, but also in assisting with the implementation of the recruitment plan. As EMR systems continue to evolve and practices continue to incorporate all parts of the medical records (laboratory, medications, visits, etc.), the entire program will become much more robust in offering assistance to the research department.

Currently, when sites answer the question of potential subjects, they usually take a guess. Unfortunately, the guess is often low or high—rarely is it right on. It is common knowledge that the number is off by about one-third. Then, the situation is made worse when sponsors review the estimate of a site's patient pool. Clinical trial managers have long seen the patient estimate as unreliable, and so they divide the number by three, four or even 10.[6]

Therefore, it is critical the site indicate from where its potential recruitment number is being derived. Current thinking continues to be seeded in

Figure 3: Investigator responses to potential study volunteers from within their practice for various studies

Indication	Dr. A	Dr. B	Dr. C	Dr. D	Dr. E	Avg.
Type II DM having had cardiac events (stroke, MI, CAD, PAD) on Metformin	200	40	2,000	150	300	538
Type II DM on Metformin only	1,000	2,000	1,500	500	2,600	1,520
Patients ages 50 to 59 who had not been vaccinated for Herpes Zoster	2,000	20,000	700	10,000	6,000	7,740
Patients ages 60 to 69 who had not been vaccinated for Herpes Zoster	6,000	2,000	600	1,000	2,000	2,230
Patients suffering from Insomnia	2,000	2,000	3,000	2,000	10,000	3,800

the idea that the number is a best guess, and therefore the mathematical calculation of only a fraction of the projected number listed is reliable. Sites must clearly articulate in the form the accuracy and confidence they have in meeting the stated enrollment target. This confidence can be assured only if sites invest adequate time and effort to ensure the information being provided is accurate. Realizing the quick turnaround expectation of these forms, it is imperative a well-managed research site have a system in place to receive, assess, answer (completely and accurately) and return these feasibilities forms within a very short window.

Perception and Reality Within the Site

During a recent case study, investigators within the same practice were shown the same study synopsis for a few different studies. They were asked how many potential study volunteers from their patient database they thought would fit the study protocol (see Figure 3). After querying the practice's EMR with the primary diagnosis of the study, the actual number of potential subjects was identified. (see Figure 4).

Clearly we can see that if the answer of such a pivotal question rests on the best guess of anyone, even the physician who sees these patients each day, the reality of meeting enrollment goals can be grossly inaccurate. Studies could be taken for which the site lacks adequate potential subjects and declined when enrollment goals easily could be met. These first steps in conducting thorough study feasibility are time and energy well spent so as to not tarnish

Figure 4: Overview of investigator averaged estimates vs. EMR actuals

Indication	Average of all the doctors	Actual numbers by EMR query	Off By	Number of wrong potential study volunteers
Type II DM having had cardiac events (stroke, MI, CAD, PAD) on Metformin	538	350	53%	188 over
Type II DM on Metformin only	1,520	4,400	65%	2,880 under
Patients ages 50 to 59 who had not been vaccinated for Herpes Zoster	7,740	4,799	61%	2,941 over
Patients ages 60 to 69 who had not been vaccinated for Herpes Zoster	2,230	3,118	26%	798 under
Patients suffering from Insomnia	3,800	1,145	232%	2,655 over

your site's reputation by becoming one of the 70% of sites that fail to meet enrollment goals.

Getting Your Message Out

Knowing that 78%[7] to 90%[8] of the public say the physician is their most trusted source of information regarding the decision of study participation, this site always chooses to first communicate from within its own database prior to reaching out to the general community. Taking this case study a step further, recruitment activity, and ultimately the actual number of randomized subjects, were measured against the potential study volunteers identified during the initial EMR query. Recruitment efforts included a layering of directed marketing activities to the pre-identified potential subject list.

First, a letter from their doctor informing them of the study opportunity was sent first-class mail on the physician's stationery, followed by a professionally designed postcard with a similar message and branded study design approximately six to eight weeks later. Additionally, similar messaging via posters and flyers was strategically placed around the office with a consistent message that had been incorporated into the letter and postcard. Attention was paid to ensure the "brand" of the study message was carried throughout all recruitment efforts to enhance study recall and study brand awareness.

Figure 5

Type of study	Percent of responses	Percent of consents obtained	Percent of randomizations	Screen failure
Vaccine	1.13%	35.85%	26.42%	9.43%
Type II Diabetes Mellitus	2.01%	57.14%	28.57%	28.57%
Hyperlipidemia	2.85%	31.58%	5.26%	26.32%
Weight loss	15.50%	16.13%	5.38%	10.75%

The studies within this case study can be categorized into two silos: disease-related clinical studies and vaccine studies. The results of the recruitment efforts can be viewed in Figure 5.

Knowing that between only 1%[9] and 4%[10] of the American population participates in clinical studies each year, coupled with the public's desire to learn about and participate in clinical studies, it is clear that targeted marketing to pre-identified subjects who have a relationship with the investigator can yield better than industry norms.

Buried within this scenario are some subtle but noteworthy recruitment best practices:

- Ensure you have a valid list of potential subjects to start the process.
- A personal letter to the potential subjects from the physician sends the message from the individual whose opinion they value.
- Use of professional stationery and personally addressing the letter to potential subjects shows respect and caring, as opposed to receiving a copied form letter.
- Creating a study brand that is carried throughout the study material reinforces the impression of the study.

And let us not forget the ability to answer the phone and schedule the appointment.

Understanding Your Target Audience

Too often, research sites are their own worst enemies when it comes to getting the word out that study opportunities exist. As is the case with any business attempting to get its message out to potential end users, in this case potential study subjects, it is critical to understand their mindset prior to entering an engagement with you. Understanding the framework they're coming from allows you to create messages that speak to potential subjects' concerns and present the information in a factual and consumable manner. All, of course, with Institutional Review Board (IRB) approval.

Ten Facts About Your Potential Study Volunteer's Perspective:

1. 94% of people recognize the importance of participating in clinical research in order to assist in the advancement of medical science.[11]
2. 75% of the general public state they have little to no knowledge about the clinical research enterprise and the participation process.[11] (CenterWatch)
3. 76% of Americans say they would be very likely or somewhat likely to participate in clinical research and 24% say they are not likely to or would not participate.[12]
4. A recent study showed less than 5% of Americans know where to find information about relevant clinical trials.[13]
5. More than 70% of those who have participated in clinical trials are likely to do so again.[14]
6. 77% of the general public say that they would consider getting involved in an appropriate clinical research study if asked.[15]
7. In a 2006 survey, 1,000 people were asked to choose which form of medical participation makes the greatest contribution to mankind. Among the options were: giving blood, volunteering in a clinical trial, raising money for a charity by running a race and donating an organ. Participating in a clinical trial finished last, with 9% of the votes.[15]
8. 44% of Americans said they viewed pharmaceutical and biotechnology companies unfavorably; 27% said they do not trust them to provide reliable information about drug side effects and safety; and 45% said they do not trust research sponsors to inform the public quickly when safety concerns about a drug are discovered.[16]
9. One in four respondents to a 2007 survey believed their doctors would expose them to unnecessary risk in clinical trials.[17]
10. The most trusted source from whom a person learns about study participation is his or her doctor.[18]

Plan, Plan and Then Plan More

After completing a thorough study feasibility process—undergoing an extensive pre-site visit followed by submitting various regulatory documents back and forth to the sponsor and ultimately to the IRB—attending investigator's meetings, completing countless hours of online training for the various systems that will be used, negotiating a budget and receiving all study supplies, thinking about recruitment is often overlooked during the study startup phase. In fact, 56% of sites report not having any recruitment plan or material submitted with their initial IRB review.[19]

A metric worth following closely is when the first study volunteer is enrolled relative to the site initiation visit and its impact on meeting enrollment targets. For sites that consent their first study volunteer within…

- 30 days = 90+% chance of meeting their enrollment target
- 60 days = 50% of meeting their enrollment target
- 90 days = <10% chance of meeting their enrollment targets[20]

The time to plan a recruitment campaign and consider the resources needed is during the feasibility period, and certainly these steps should be completed prior to agreeing to participate. The saying "Fool me once shame on you, fool me twice shame on me" is all too well being incorporated within our industry fabric. Do not allow your site to be one of those uninvited to receive future study opportunities due to poor past performance. Take the time to plan the recruitment campaign and be sure to execute it and measure your results.

Thirty-Seven or Twenty-Two

Think of companies that make you feel special. What do they do? I doubt it's high-ticket items or constant attention. In fact, I'll bet it's about the way you're treated when you're in their presence, and perhaps a small but meaningful token of appreciation following that encounter more than anything else. It takes 37 muscles to frown and only 22 to smile—sometimes less really is more.

All data point to the fact that those engaged in a clinical trial believe it to be a positive experience and would highly consider participating again. Clearly that decision is multifactorial; however, the manner in which volunteers are treated during a study carries a strong indication of their willingness to sign up for the next study. That experience ends with informing subjects of the study's outcome. Be sure to remember this small but very important aspect of their study participation by letting them know what arm they were randomized to during the study and the results.

Creating a Culture of Appreciation

To conclude, here are 10 ideas sites have shared that can be considered outside-the-box thinking to help create a culture of appreciation. All are easily implementable with a little effort.

1. Remember study volunteers' special days with a card—for their birthday or their anniversary of joining the study;
2. Ask their opinion at the end of the study—a short survey of their experience;
3. Invite study volunteers to a Halloween party—have staff dress up and serve the food (also invite other office staff as a way to incorporate them into the research department's efforts);
4. Host an annual research luncheon;
5. Keep volunteers informed—mail a regularly scheduled newsletter about study opportunities and information about clinical research in general;
6. Wall of Appreciation—take their pictures and place them on a wall with a banner saying "Thank You To Our Study Volunteers" (you will need signed waivers to post their pictures);
7. Invite study volunteers to a summer cookout;
8. Provide each study volunteer with a certificate of appreciation;
9. Provide snacks and reading material during their visits;
10. Be sincere and genuine—nothing goes further than people knowing you really care!

Author Biography

Christine Pierre is the founder, president and CEO of RxTrials, Inc. She is internationally known for her experience and expertise in clinical research site management and patient recruitment and retention for the clinical trials industry. For the past 20 years Christine has been providing site management services to research sites in all types of settings, education, operation and clinical expertise, and training and consultation services to sponsors and CROs. Christine's understanding of the clinical research site's processes allows her to work with sites and sponsors/CROs to help expedite the clinical research recruitment process by bringing in study volunteers in a timely and efficient manner and providing high-quality research data. Christine created The RxTrials Institute (RxTi) to offer training and education through both public and customized courses to research professionals. She is also the founder and host of the Site Solutions Summit, an industry conference that identifies and establishes best business practices for sites. Christine is a frequent speaker at industry conferences, and served as chair of the Association of Clinical Research Professionals (ACRP) in 2008, an editorial board member of Clinical Trials Advisor and eCliniqua, a steering committee member of the Clinical Trials Transformation Initiative (CTTI), and a board of advisors member for both the Center for Information & Study on Clinical Research

(CISCRP) and Hands Across the Americas. In 2009, PharmaVOICE named Christine one of the "100 Most Inspiring People" in the life sciences industry. She was named a Woman of the Year by the National Association of Professional Women for 2011-12. Christine is currently completing her second book on clinical research site management.

References

1. U.S. Department of Health and Human Services, Office of Inspector General, "Challenges to FDA's Ability to Monitor and Inspect Foreign Clinical Trials," OIG, June 2010.
2. The Site Investigator Questionnaire, RxTrials, 2009.
3. The Site Solutions Summit Survey, 2010.
4. The Tufts Center for the Study of Drug Development, Outlook 2006.
5. Bio/Pharmaceutical R&D Statistical Sourceboook 2009/2010, Parexel International.
6. Harper, B and Zuckerman, D., "No Virginia, There is No Enrollment Problem: Bursting the Myth of Late Enrollment," *The Monitor*, October 2008.
7. Centerwatch Surveys, 2007–2009.
8. "The Will and Why Survey," BBK Healthcare/Harris Interactive, June 2001; Public Perception Survey, RxTrials.
9. Health Day News, posted online 4/1/08.
10. The Center for Information and Study on Clinical Research Participation (CISCRP), Facts & Figures, 2011.
11. CenterWatch.
12. Research!America's "America Speaks, Poll Data Summary," 2010.
13. Getz, K., 2004. Survey of 1,170 adults at the Clinical Trial Congress in Philadelphia, Penn., Institute for International Research, February 2004.
14. Raskob, G., and Hotez, P., "Sometimes bumpy road pays large dividends for health," *Edmond Sun*, June 4, 2008.
15. CISCRP, www.ciscrp.org.
16. Kaiser Foundation, 2008.
17. Braunstein, *Medicine*, 2008.
18. Harris Interactive Will & Why Survey, RxTrials Public Perception Survey.

19. The Site Solutions Summit Survey, 2010.
20. AAiPharma, 2005.

CHAPTER TWELVE

New Technology for Global Patient Retention

By Melynda Geurts, M.S.

Retention, by simple definition, is the capacity or power to retain. In relation to clinical trials, patient retention is the sponsor's ability to create an environment that maintains constant engagement among trial participants to yield statistically significant study outcomes.

In 2010, an article in *Life Science Leader* titled, "Importance of Patient Retention Strategies," stated that 30% of phase III trial participants dropped out.[1] In the last decade, attrition has increased by 36%; a study conducted by Tufts Center for the Study of Drug Development suggests that this is a growing trend.[2] These high dropout rates can invalidate clinical trial data, resulting in unacceptable findings by global regulatory agencies.[3] Therefore, recruitment and retention must be executed in concert to minimize potential long-range costs associated with extending enrollment to counter unplanned attrition rates.

As the clinical research industry advances, identifying, recruiting and retaining study participants grows more complex. Several phenomena intensify the urgency to retain subjects in clinical trials, including increased competition among trial sponsors, emergence of personalized medicine, certain patient populations based on age and mobility, protocol complexities and trial procedures, declining trial participation and establishment of the Health Insurance Portability and Accountability Act (HIPAA). The overall duration of clinical trials has increased by 74%.[4] Likewise, HIPAA regulations and guidelines impose significant time and cost burdens on researchers.[5]

Apart from the inherent challenges associated with protocol complexities and federal regulations, the industry's silo approach to conducting clinical trials impedes patient retention. Most often sponsors focus on the cost of delays if a study does not finish on time. What about the cost of delays that occur when actual dropout rates far exceed projected attrition and enrollment must be re-engaged?

"Attempting to rebuild a depleted patient cohort with replacements midstream may be cost prohibitive and logistically cumbersome," said Scott H. Connor, vice president of marketing for Acurian. As a result, many study managers proactively implement retention programs to mitigate the unforeseen costs of lost patients.[3]

Dropout rates and non-adherence are pervasive problems in clinical research. On one hand, there are retention challenges due to study design. On the other are the growing societal demands that hinder one's ability to maintain study compliance given personal time limitations. Even studies with multiple retention techniques may experience low retention rates.[6] Therefore, the emerging model of participant retention in clinical research will require providers to advance their solutions beyond traditional retention methods. Consumer and provider sophistication must coincide. To make this happen, we must understand the "new" study participant.

Consumer vs. Patient Approach

The turn of the 21st century ushered in a boon in internet use, more specifically, social media. Global access to the internet makes an infinite amount of information readily available at any time. This phenomenon has changed the way individuals receive information and manage their personal health. It has also changed the way individuals engage with their physicians and healthcare communities.

In this changing landscape, individuals who participate in clinical trials are shifting from passive participants (i.e., research "subjects") to active participants (e.g.,research "volunteers" or "consumers").[7] They are claiming their place as consumers within the clinical trial process, resulting in higher expectations with respect to trial outcomes, site accommodations and staff-to-patient communication. They expect to have 24/7 online access to relevant study information before, during and after trial participation. Additionally, trial consumers expect the communication lines to be two-way.[8] They do not just want information filtered to them; rather, they demand the option to initiate contact with study staff as needed.

Since its inception, the clinical research industry has been challenged with enhancing public knowledge about the clinical trial proces in an effort to generate interest and raise enrollment. To reinvigorate this effort, the industry must reevaluate its approach to recruitment and its perception of patient populations. Viewing study participants as consumers rather than subjects will engender heightened focus on patient education and customer service principles which will, in turn, promote patient satisfaction and continued study participation. In a CenterWatch survey of 670 study volunteers, 91% of respondents said they would participate in a clinical trial again if given the opportunity. This response shows that once patients learn of trials and participate in them, the experience is positive. It makes the case for modifying our educational process. Setting the right stage up front will result in committed participation.

According to a report by the Center for Information and Study on Clinical Research Participation (CISCRP), "If instruction is linked to personal contact, potential volunteers will be better equipped to make informed decisions and remain confident throughout the trial. Further education must extend initial connections between volunteers and the center to ensure their overall satisfaction and to encourage their sustained involvement as participants and advocates."[7]

CISCRP conducted a series of focus groups among 22 study volunteers to determine what factors most inform and educate clinical research participants. One outcome of these focus groups was the identification of a core set of motivations of all study volunteers, regardless of age and socioeconomic status. "These motivations serve as a blueprint for patient and public education and outreach. Study volunteers want to:

- feel they are taking control of their medical condition and well-being
- develop personal relationships with study staff
- be treated as human beings
- know that their participation will make a difference."[7]

Given limited research literacy among the public, it is the industry's responsibility to manage expectations of trial consumers so they understand the purpose of research, feel confident about participation, are inspired to consider subsequent studies and, most importantly, are compelled to tell others about their experiences. No different than with product marketing, a consumer will tell five to seven people if they are unhappy about a product he purchased but will tell only three to four people if he is satisfied. We must, therefore, focus on ensuring a positive experience to avoid the short-term ramifications and instead reap long-term benefits from word-of-mouth advertising.

Setting the stage to manage trial consumers' expectations is key to yielding committed participants. However, retention and education do not stop when the study concludes. Pre- and post-trial education must meet trial consumers' needs and expectations. "The post-trial follow-up is a pivotal moment when research centers can reinforce the relationships built before and during the study volunteer's enrollment period," according to a CISCRP report. "Education provided after a trial's conclusion will benefit the growing populations of volunteers clamoring for information, while strengthening the research center's backbone of satisfied, active participants."[7]

Figure 1 illustrates CISCRP's model for providing participants the education, enthusiasm and support they need to become ambassadors of the clinical research process. This model should be adapted by all who participate in the clinical research space and directly interact with trial consumers.[9]

Managing expectations is just one part of the equation. There are other factors that influence trial consideration and continuation, including logistical, physical, educational, emotional and outside influencers such as family members, friends and personal doctors. Several studies have investigated the demographic, behavioral and psychological characteristics of individuals who discontinue trial participation. For example, younger participants

Figure 1: CISCRP's model for success

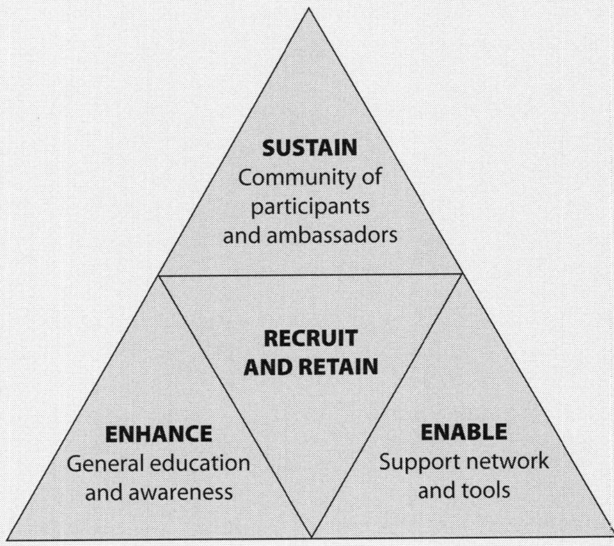

Source: CISCRP

tend to discontinue more often than older participants. One explanation for this is that younger participants face numerous family demands and obligations that may not affect older individuals.[6] Conversely, older participants may be faced with declining health problems and, therefore, are motivated to continue their study participation. Other demographic influences include ethnicity, education and employment status. Psychological and behavioral deterrents include depression, psychological distress, substance abuse, hostility and negative attitudes about healthcare.

In addition to evaluating the characteristics of individuals who chose to withdraw from research studies, CISCRP analyzed the reasons for withdrawal as stated by study volunteers. The most frequently cited reasons were competing work-life obligations, logistical challenges such as unreliable transportation or inflexible study visit schedules, study demands (e.g., patient diaries and reporting procedures) and lack of motivation or commitment. Of these, work-life responsibilities ranked highest.[6]

Understanding trial consumers' expectations, motivations and demographic/psychological profiles is pivotal for averting attrition and maintaining momentum throughout the clinical trial paradigm—before, during and after. Hence, educating and engaging study volunteers has become more "patient-centric" than ever before. Novel technological solutions are in high demand to support retention initiatives.

Novel Strategies to Enhance Global Retention

Ensuring a successful trial experience among study volunteers requires a proactive retention and education program that focuses on marketing to the site's own patients, establishing communication efficiencies and giving volunteers a reason to return. To achieve these goals, many companies have proactively built global retention into their business models. Other organizations have added this strategy to their repertoire in response to market demands. Organizations taking on the patient retention challenge include patient recruitment and retention companies, CROs and niche service providers.

Contract Research Organizations (CROs)

If the medical research industry hopes to expand and strengthen its participant base, building and maintaining a community of volunteers, researchers, physicians and other study staff will be necessary. According to CISCRP, "Constant communication, through conversations between volunteers and study personnel, informational forums for participants in specific trials and post-trial resources will ensure that volunteers stay aware of ongoing study opportunities and feel more than a transitory connection to clinical research. Investing in personal relationships—between volunteers and their study staff or other participants—is a pivotal element in successful education."[7] This foundation fostered the creation of online communities among clinical research providers.

For illustration purposes, the online communities of PPD and Quintiles will be highlighted. PPD is a global CRO providing drug discovery, development and lifecycle management services to the clinical research industry. In March 2011, PPD unveiled its online portal, PatientView, linking clinical trial participants with biopharmaceutical firms, physicians and healthcare resources to improve patient connectivity in clinical trials. PatientView is customizable, allows patients online access to valuable health information and is a convenient way to stay in continual contact with the trial registry and monitoring program.

Quintiles is a fully integrated service provider offering clinical, commercial, consulting and capital solutions. Quintiles operates ClinicalResearch.com, an online community to increase the awareness of, understanding of and participation in clinical research studies. This online community supports all potentially involved parties in clinical research, including healthy volunteers, patients, caregivers, physicians and health professionals. Individuals may opt-in to become part of the database to receive ongoing communications about clinical trial opportunities based on the information they provide.

These are just two examples of many online communities that exist to address the growing demand for real-time, constant communication among various clinical research entities and trial consumers.

Patient Recruitment and Retention Organizations (PROs)

PROs are also making inroads addressing the demands for information and support among trial consumers. In response, companies such as DAC Patient Recruitment Services (DAC) have specialized training programs, and others (such as Acurian and MediciGlobal) have created and launched technology platforms.

DAC is a comprehensive patient recruitment, retention and training provider in the clinical trials industry. As a certified continuing education provider, DAC is able to establish and enhance the communication platform desired and needed by volunteers with study personnel. This platform is created through highly-targeted, study-specific training conducted among a study's research staff (i.e., CRCs, CRAs, PIs). This hands-on service offering is proven to increase enrollment activity by 30% within 30 days of training in some instances. In the case of retention, the awareness building generated by training activities is highly measurable based on outcomes directly tracked and related to training content, with as much as a 50% decrease in attrition measured within 30 days of a global training program, for example.

Acurian is a full-service provider of clinical trial patient recruitment and retention solutions for the life sciences industry. In 2010, it launched a technology platform called Retention Manager™, innovative, comprehensive software with an array of direct services to support patient retention. According to a 2010 industry white paper by Scott H. Connor, "Retention Manager™ generates a constant stream of communication within the system and between the patient and the site coordinator so that each knows what the next step is and what steps have already been taken."[3]

In June 2011, Acurian launched a new clinical trial patient education platform to assist sites in helping volunteers better understand their participation in research studies and manage their expectations. The platform consists of videos customized for each trial, including informed consent and patient engagement modules. All educational elements can be shown in the physician's office, viewed via iPhone or iPad and delivered to the volunteer's email.[11]

MediciGlobal is a patient recruitment-retention specialty firm serving the clinical trials industry. Addressing rising attrition rates and the number of volunteers that become lost-to-follow-up became the company's focus. To address this, MediciGlobal created a specific lost-to-follow-up program called L2FU™, which features the following components:

- Proactive development and implementation of patient retention programs
- Recovery of patients already lost-to-follow-up
- Ongoing just-in-time lost-to-follow-up.

PROs are rapidly developing new, yet unique, approaches within the clinical trial process to target key areas identified as ongoing challenges. Online technology creates another touch point with trial consumers, serving their highest need.

Niche Service Organizations

Successful trial completion can occur only if the targeted number of enrolled volunteers stays engaged and completes the study. Without an adequate sample size, there can be no analysis to prove the safety and efficacy of investigational products. Mobile technology has emerged as a viable tool to enhance patient retention. In a recent Nielsen poll, 79% of individuals between ages 12 and 65+ said they communicated by text message more often than by phone.

Figure 2: Number of calls vs. SMS sent/received per month

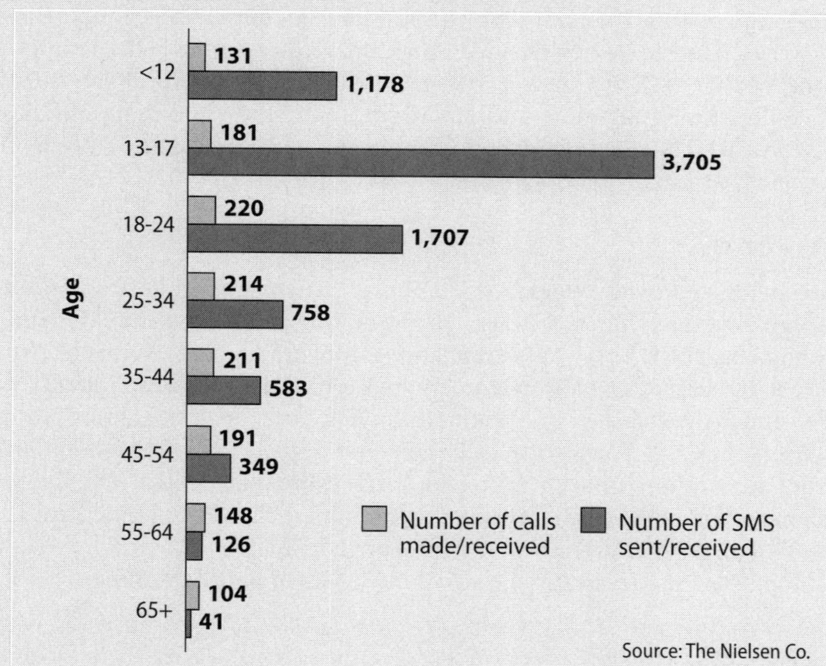

This trend has prompted the development and refinement of niche service providers within the life sciences industry, including Clinical Trial Media (CTM), Exco InTouch, HealthCentral and Greenphire. All have developed innovative technology solutions to help combat the rise in attrition.

Clinical Trial Media (CTM)

CTM is a full-service, global patient recruitment and retention firm specializing in patient outreach headquartered in Jericho, N.Y. Early on, CTM recognized the need and importance of creating and maintaining frequent communication between the study team and volunteers to keep them engaged. Understanding the cost implications of volunteers who drop out of a study or are non-compliant, CTM focused on creating a system to transform the mobile phone into a robust retention and compliance tool.

According to a report issued by the United Nations, there are more than 4.6 million mobile cellular subscriptions worldwide. The same report recognized the importance of the cell phone in healthcare, particularly in the developing world. The messaging system created by CTM allows volunteers who have opted in to receive text message reminders for appointments, dosing, diary compliance and other events essential to keep patients compliant and committed. The system also allows motivational messages to be sent, enabling patients to immediately text or call back the site to reschedule appointments, for example. CTM's system operates anywhere in the world and in the trial consumer's local language.

Legions of Smartphones, iPhones and other mobile devices support applications that can be downloaded providing greater functionality than text alone. At the touch of a button, volunteers can see their entire appointment schedules, dosing regimens and other important study information. Using this level of technology provides trial consumers with the highest amount of flexibility, a trait highly sought after.[13]

Exco InTouch

Exco InTouch provides regulatory-compliant patient management solutions. Recognizing that effective site-patient communication is essential to maintaining engagement and full compliance throughout a study, Exco InTouch has led the adaptation of mobile technology for this very purpose. Like CTM, Exco InTouch considers cell phone technology the global communication method of choice. Worldwide, cell phone use outpaces landline use and internet access approximately four-fold.[14] And more than 70% of cell phones are owned in developing countries,[14] meaning high levels of immediate access to patients within trials—regardless of geography.

Mobile technology is the gateway to the future of patient retention.

Figure 3: Characteristics that make the mobile platform effective in patient retention and compliance

- Discrete, unobtrusive for sensitive scenarios
- Integrates easily into volunteer's life
- Familiar, simple and easy to use
- Ubiquitous technology, supports global trials
- Device independent, SMS is standard functionality
- Portable, providing immediate access (24/7)
- Real-time communication
- Phone ownership increases care taken
- Cost neutral to patients and sites

Source: Exco InTouch, 2011.

The following case study further illustrates the impact mobile technology can have on patient retention and compliance.

Case Study

Study characteristics

- Global vaccine study—13 countries
- SMS reminder services used in six countries
- 21 sites and 2,566 volunteers

Figure 4: Case study outcomes comparing site performance based on SMS services adoption

Background	13 countries selected for the study. SMS services were used in six countries covering 21 sites and 2,566 patients
Global results	Sites participating in SMS service saw 94% reduction in discontinuation compared with non-SMS sites
Country example	The following results are for sites based in the U.S.: · 10% of SMS sites had discontinuation, compared with 90% of non-SMS sites · 62% of SMS sites had visits within visit window, compared with 7% of non-SMS sites · 94% of subjects using SMS services were within visit window, compared with 79% of non-SMS subjects

HealthCentral

HealthCentral is a network of more than 35 interactive health sites whose mission is to empower millions of people to improve and take control of their health and well-being. HealthCentral predicted that consumers would eventually forego specific web sites and instead seek health information via their preferred internet search engine. As a result, HealthCentral focuses on enhancing search engine optimization via the creation of unique quality content most often sought by consumers.

Unlike a portal, through which a volunteer might go to a home page to seek information on one topic and then be distracted by something entirely unrelated, volunteers coming to HealthCentral typically arrive via so-called "long tail searches" (of three or more words related to a specific question) on search engines. As a result, these individuals have identified themselves as seeking content related to their own or a loved one's health journey. Manhattan Research's annual Cybercitizen survey found that about 60% of online consumers with a chronic condition—and two-thirds of online caregivers—are electronically empowered.

What is an "empowered consumer"? In February to March 2010, the University of Virginia surveyed 2,888 patients in cooperation with HealthCentral regarding online behavior. The study found empowered consumers are far more likely to seek other patients' experiences and share their own. They also are more likely to make a healthcare post via social media such as Facebook and/or tweet on a healthcare issue. Of those surveyed, 30% were considered empowered and 50% were deemed "traditional mainstream," available to be elevated into the empowered group by intellectual arguments and social influence.

HealthCentral uses Clinical Trial Recruitment Centers to create online communities to engage individuals searching for information on a specific disease. The ongoing, up-to-date information that is continually channeled through the Clinical Trial Recruitment Center is the glue that keeps the empowered consumer connected. For example, HealthCentral used a Recruitment Center to reach individuals with heart valve disease. The goal was to identify and recruit 75 qualified referrals within three and a half months. HealthCentral identified 90 qualified referrals in two and a half months using its online community platform.

Leveraging an online community is like throwing a neighborhood cocktail party: You must first nurture a trusted relationship over time before expecting people to show up. Leveraging existing disease-specific communities and recruiting volunteers actively seeking treatment options is far faster and more efficient than traditional media recruitment methods, according to HealthCentral.[15]

Greenphire

Greenphire is a leading provider of clinical payment and communication technology solutions. Recognizing longstanding deficiencies in traditional clinical trial payment and communication methods, Greenphire developed web-based solutions to streamline the arduous (and expensive) task of efficiently administering clinical trials. Its best-known web-based solution is its ClinCard System. The ClinCard System is a globally deployable, web-based patient payment, patient management and patient communication platform that has emerged as an innovative alternative to conventional systems.

The ClinCard System enables study administrators (at sites and sponsors) to deliver patient payments, including stipend and travel reimbursements, to the patient in real time and allows the patient to gain immediate access to funds as he/she completes a visit or other study milestone. Patients receive a MasterCard debit card uniquely branded with the study logo. The system allows the administrators to oversee and approve all payments and communications across their site or study from a central web portal and access a suite of reports to facilitate accounting, compliance and documentation throughout the trial.

Programs using the ClinCard System have recorded a significant impact in subject retention. In a recent case study in which the ClinCard System was implemented as a rescue strategy for half of the total enrolled patients

Figure 5: Study retention rate comparison

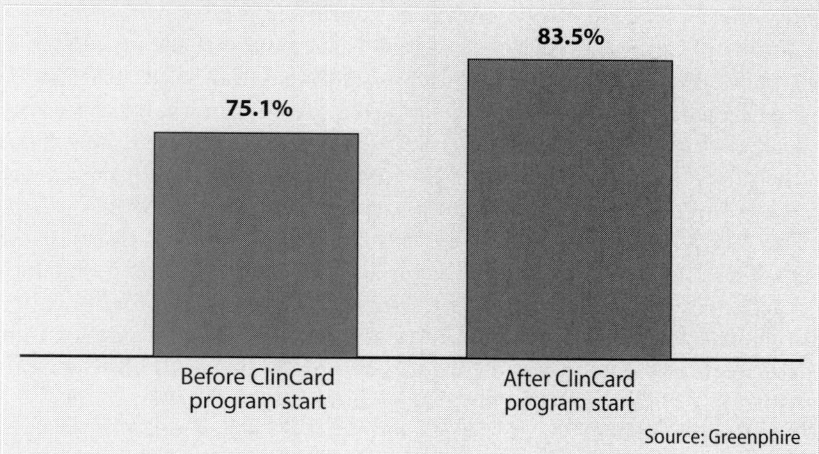

Figure 6: Cumulative attrition by visit

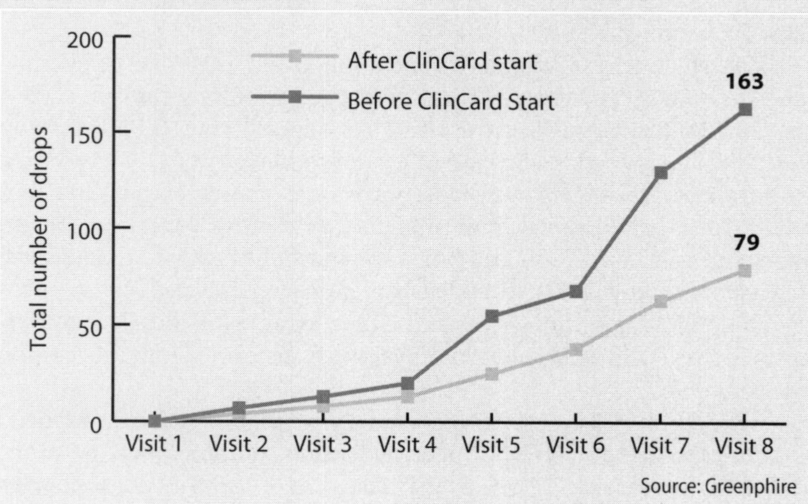

(2,552), retention in the ClinCard test group increased by 11.2% over the non-ClinCard group. The value of retention was realized most drastically as the time between visits increased in the later stages of the study.

By leveraging new technology to streamline patient payments and communication, the ClinCard System has improved the patient experience throughout a study and encouraged a new, patient-centric model in the clinical trial environment.[16]

Pharmaceutical Companies

Lastly, select pharmaceutical companies are raising the bar with the implementation of novel approaches to address participation challenges. Pfizer recently announced FDA approval to conduct a virtual trial called the REMOTE study. Participants in this study will not be required to come in for office visits. Instead, they will use mobile phones and web-based technology to collect data on the safety and efficacy of Detrol LA (tolterodine tartrate), Pfizer's extended-release investigational treatment for overactive bladder (OAB).

The REMOTE study aims to recruitment 600 volunteers from 10 U.S. states. The study has the potential to broaden the available trial populations and accelerate clinical development, while cutting costs, improving patient compliance, reducing withdrawal rates and delivering better-quality, more reliable real-time data. Additionally, this effort is in line with improving the transparency of clinical trials and the resulting data to trial consumers.[17]

"Studies like REMOTE could make biomedical science much more accessible to people who have long been excluded from or under-represented in clinical trials," said Dr. Freda Lewis-Hall, Pfizer's executive vice president and chief medical officer. "Putting research within reach of more diverse populations has the potential to advance medical progress and lead to better outcomes for more patients."[18]

This level of trial conduct consideration could potentially catapult a change in how the industry manages global retention programs in chronic, long-term conditions such as overactive bladder (as in the REMOTE study), Type 2 diabetes, hypertension, and other indications.

In summary, the industry still faces annual rise of attrition rates in clinical trials. Industry professionals have undergone extensive education to better understand trial consumers and how to manage their expectations to yield desired participation levels. Providers have quickly capitalized on this knowledge by developing technology-based educational platforms. Through this transition, the traditional study volunteer has transformed into the "empowered" volunteer.

As we move into the next decade, data collection and outcome reporting will continue to grow in importance. Retention solutions must be nimble to meet the ever-changing needs and demands of the trial consumer. The industry can meet these challenges by embracing and innovating technology solutions.

Author Biography

Melynda Geurts has presented at numerous conferences and seminars worldwide in the clinical trials industry. As vice president of operations at DAC Patient Recruitment Services, an Imperial company, her influence is instrumental to business development, contract negotiations, project operations and site management. Geurts was a contributing writer for Diana Anderson's "*A Guide to Patient Recruitment*" and "*A Guide to Patient Recruitment and Retention.*" In 2008, *PharmaVOICE* magazine named her one of the "100 Most Inspiring People in the Life-Sciences Industry."

References

1. Elvidge, Suzannne. *Importance of Patient Retention Strategies.* Life Science Leader, 2010.
2. Kaitin, KI. *Growing Protocol Design Complexity Stresses Investigators, Volunteers.* Impact Report 2008.
3. Connor, Scott H. (2010). *An Integrated Approach for Clinical Trial Patient Retention.* [White paper]. Retrieved from www.ngpsummit.com/media/whitepapers/Acurian_Retention_NGPUS.pdf
4. Connor, Scott H. *Keeping Patients in Clinical Trials.* Drug Discovery & Development. 2011; Available at: www.dddmag.com/article-Keeping-Patients-in-Clinical-Trials-2711.aspx. Accessed April 1, 2011.
5. *Addressing Clinical Trial Recruitment and Patient Retention Issues Imposed by HIPAA Step by Step (third of a series).* Lost To Follow-Up. 2008; Available at: http://lost-to-follow-up.com/patient-retention. Accessed April 1, 2011.
6. Gonder-Frederick Ph.D., Linda. *Participant Retention in Clinical Research: A Major Challenge.* University of Virginia School of Medicine Improving Control with Activity and Nutrition. Spring 2008; Available at: www.healthsystem.virginia.edu/internet/ican/lgf_spring_08.doc. Accessed April 1, 2011.
7. *Factors That Most Inform and Educate Clinical Research Participants.* CISCRP. Available at: www.ciscrp.org/professional/concerns.html. Accessed April 1, 2011.
8. *Enhanced Involvement of Clinical Trial Patients Results in Lower Drop-Out Rates.* Study Portal. Available at: www.clinicaltrial-portal.com/services/patient-retention-tools. Accessed April 1, 2011.
9. Simmons, Diane, and Getz, Kenneth. *What Patients Expect, Need, and Want to Know about Clinical Research*; Global Forum; October 2010; Vol. 2, Issue 5.
10. Pharmaceutical Business Review. *PPD Unveils New Technology Portal for Patient Retention in Clinical Trials.* PBR. March 10, 2010. Available at: http://itsoftware.pharmaceutical-business-review.com/news/ppd-unveils-new-technology-portal-for-patient-retention-in-clinical-trials-100311. Accessed April 1, 2011.
11. Connor, Scott H. *Acurian Announces New Clinical Trial Patient Education Platform.* Genetic Engineering & Biotechnology News. June 2, 2011. Available at: www.genengnews.com/industry-updates/acurian-

announces-new-clinical-trial-patient-education-platform/119467011. Accessed June 9, 2011.

12. *Lost 2 Follow Up*. MediciGlobal. http://mediciglobal.com/services/category/global_patient_retention. Accessed June 14, 2011.
13. *Patient Retention and the Power of Mobile Devices*. Clinical Trial Media. May 2011.
14. ITU—The World in 2010.
15. *Empowered Patient Internet Usage.* HealthCentral. May 2011
16. *New Modalities in Clinical Trial Payments for Patients*. Greenphire. May 2011.
17. Mansell, Peter. *Pfizer Announces 'Virtual' Clinical Trial Pilot in US.* PharmaTimes. June 9, 2011. Available at: www.pharmatimes.com/article/11-06-09/Pfizer_announces_virtual_clinical_trial_pilot_in_US.aspx. Accessed June 14, 2011.

CHAPTER THIRTEEN

Case Study of a Global Trial: Challenges and Solutions in Execution and Delivery

By Lacey Powers

Each new global recruitment or retention program presents a unique opportunity for learning. As country regulations change and study teams have increasing acceptance for recruitment strategies, there is an ever-present and ever-growing list of lessons learned. New knowledge affords more effective and more tailored recruitment programs and ultimately higher return on investment for sponsors. The following case study reflects a recently completed global recruitment program by DAC Patient Recruitment Services for a multiple sclerosis trial. This program, containing only ex-U.S. sites and quite a diverse assortment of strategies, proved to be a breeding ground for lessons learned.

Objectives

- Understand the components of this global patient recruitment program.
- Identify challenges in implementing global recruitment initiatives.
- Develop processes that facilitate smooth global execution.
- Understand the importance of tracking outcomes of program initiatives.

Case Study Specifics

- A multi-center, randomized study comparing the effectiveness and safety of the IP to the standard of care in patients with relapsing multiple sclerosis

- 300 patients
- 46 investigative sites
- Duration of study participation was approximately one year
- Inclusion/exclusion criteria were in line with other multiple sclerosis trials, and there were no specific outliers or criteria that made enrollment particularly difficult
- Target enrollment period was 18 months
- 13 total countries participated in the study. At program initiation, the following 10 countries were included: Germany, Canada, France, Hungary, Italy, Poland, Spain, Tunisia, Greece and Czech Republic. Over the course of the program, Belgium, the U.K. and Switzerland were added.

Program Elements

Kick-off Meeting

The kick-off meeting was a face-to-face meeting held at the sponsor's offices. The date was scheduled immediately following execution of the contract, and the sponsor attendees included various directors, the clinical trial manager and the clinical trial assistant. Discussions highlighted timelines for the study's recruitment program design, development and implementation and assignment of responsibilities. The description of services was described in detail, and potential recruitment challenges were discussed. This face-to-face meeting allowed the teams an opportunity to establish a positive working relationship to enhance delivery of the recruitment program.

Study Branding and Messaging

To achieve maximum awareness of the study, DAC created an easily identifiable study brand used on correspondence to the patient community, the medical community and study personnel. This was an easy-to-identify graphic logo design that accompanied the study name.

DAC generated a study message/concept targeted to patients as well as a separate message that targeted physicians. Each message included a blend of important trial information with an eye-catching design so it would stand out. The messaging elements were carried through all of the patient and physician materials.

Site Needs Research Survey

To understand the past experiences at each site related to effective recruitment strategies, DAC reached out to all sites with an electronic survey. The approximate completion time was less than 10 minutes. The purpose of the survey was to open a dialog between DAC and the sites and to assess the following areas:

- Acceptance of the recruitment program elements
- Proper routing of external patient referrals
- Contact information to be printed on recruitment materials
- Past strategies that proved effective for similar studies
- Expected recruitment challenges related to this trial
- Additional thoughts related to the trial or recruitment program.

DAC compiled this information and provided it to the appropriate sponsor team members. This included in-house team members as well as those in the field in each country. The information was used to customize the approach to each site and to provide a different perspective to the sponsor related to the site needs and challenges with recruitment. The survey findings were used as ongoing discussion for dialog during the Country Program Lead/CRA teleconferences.

Surveys were sent to a total of 65 sites, 50 of which completed them.

Online Recruitment Training Module for Sites

To have a detailed explanation of the recruitment program available to sites at all times, DAC created a presentation of the recruitment program elements that was uploaded into an online module. This module was maintained by the sponsor, and user IDs and passwords were distributed to sites prior to initiation. The module was stored alongside other modules for which completion was mandatory. The training module ensured exposure to the recruitment program at every investigative site.

Recruitment Training for Country Project Leads (CPLs) and CRAs

At the onset of the program, and prior to launching the program to the sites, DAC conducted two webcasts to present the recruitment program to the country leads and CRAs. The success of the program was contingent on support from these key team members, as they were directly interfacing with the investigative sites. DAC facilitated the webcasts; however, the sponsor's management team delivered the welcome message to the attendees and encouraged the teams in each country to support the recruitment program.

Bi-monthly CPL and CRA Recruitment Teleconferences

DAC developed and facilitated 30-minute teleconferences with the country leads and CRAs every other month for the duration of the recruitment period. The teleconferences included a short recruitment strategy learning session, a study-specific lessons learned/best practices segment and an open-forum discussion on how to enhance usage of the recruitment initiatives/materials available to the study sites. Based on screening activity tracked in IVRS, DAC identified sites that had no recent screening activity, and these sites were discussed in detail during these teleconferences. These calls created action items for the country teams, to encourage activity at sites that did not seem engaged in the study. Attendance was kept at a maximum of three countries per call, to avoid lengthy site-specific discussions that would have been irrelevant to other countries. These teleconferences were designed to maintain ongoing focus and accountability for study enrollment and the recruitment support available to the study sites.

DAC completed a total of 26 teleconferences with the country leads and CRAs.

Recruitment Kits

DAC developed recruitment kits/materials that were provided to study sites. These materials gave the sites critical awareness-building materials that allowed them to introduce the study to patients within the investigative sites and also within the surrounding community. Materials were translated into the appropriate languages for all countries that participated in the trial, with the exception of Greece. Materials (and quantities) provided to the sites included:

- Two self-standing study posters
- 50 fliers
- 10 patient education booklets
- One brochure holder
- One recruitment kit box

DAC shipped a total of 56 recruitment kits to sites.

Site Toolkits

To support the investigative sites with screening and patient identification, DAC created tool kits containing reference materials for the study teams. Each kit was shipped to the appropriate CRA for each site, prior to the site's initiation. The contents of the kit included:

- Two physician-focused study posters for internal use
- Three pocket protocols
- 10 inclusion/exclusion cards

- 50 pre-screening worksheets
- One study procedure quick-reference flip book

Materials in the toolkits were provided in English only, and kits were sent to 100% of the sites participating in the trial.

Physician-to-Patient Mailers

Sites were encouraged to use their existing database of patients to generate a list of potential patients for this trial. DAC provided appropriate materials that could be mailed to patients as an introduction to the trial. These materials included:

- Physician-to-patient letter
- Patient-focused study brochure
- Branded study magnet with the study URL

These packages were sent in bulk to the investigative sites with return mailing labels affixed. Sites were required to include the patient's name, mailing address and postage.

A total of 2,300 patient mailings were sent to sites. These were mailed to patients and/or distributed to patients in a clinic setting.

Community Outreach

DAC identified organizations supporting MS patients within most countries participating in the trial. The main organization targeted was the lead MS society, which exists in most countries. Greece was not targeted with community outreach strategies, as this type of outreach to patients is not permitted. DAC reached out to the various organizations by phone and email to assess opportunities to build trial awareness within the MS community. DAC presented study information in both electronic and hard copy. The goal was to reach MS patients directly, and this was achieved through work with support groups, patient newsletters and online trial listings that linked to the study-specific web site.

International Study Web Site

One of the most significant components of this recruitment program was the international study-specific web site. This was a key vehicle for directly accessing the target population in each country. DAC's proposal included design, development and programming and hosting of the study web site. The web site included six patient-focused pages and provided:

- An overview of the study

- Education on clinical research in general
- Answers to frequently asked questions
- A site locator
- A pre-screening option

The online pre-screening function allowed patients to identify as a potential/appropriate study participant for the trial. The pre-screener consisted of 16 questions a patient could answer to determine whether he or she met high-level eligibility criteria and could be contacted by a site for further screening. The questions included items such as age, diagnosis, relapse history and medical history. Overall, the questions included in the pre-screener were developed through collaboration between DAC and the sponsor. There was some slight variation in the pre-screener within each country, based on what type of information was permissible to collect from a patient.

The countries in which web sites were launched included:

- Spain
- Poland
- U.K.
- Belgium (Dutch and French)
- Tunisia (Arabic and French)

The pre-screening report and contact information for those individuals who qualified through the process were forwarded directly to the appropriate site, and a blinded referral notification email was sent to DAC. The notification email allowed DAC to track referrals and follow up with sites regarding patient status on final outcome. All web site users were provided the contact information for the investigative site that was to receive the pre-screening report. This allowed the initial contact to come from either the patient or the site.

In Spain, the ethics authorities would not permit collection of the patient's contact information. To comply with this regulation, when a patient "passed" pre-screening, he or she was assigned a unique identification number. This number was then forwarded to the site along with the screening report. The patient was instructed to make note of that identification number and to reference it when contacting the site. Logistically, this process worked well and was permitted by the EC as an acceptable alternative.

Web Marketing

DAC marketed the study web site through a regionalized pay-per-click campaign within each country, based on the location of the investigative sites.

Physician-to-Physician Education Packages

DAC deployed an educationally-based physician outreach program targeting neurologists within an approximate 50-mile radius of the investigative sites. This program was designed to help establish and maintain flow of external patient referrals. DAC developed a packet of physician-focused materials to educate physicians with information regarding the trial design and the investigational product. Packages were suitable for direct mailings and/or distribution to an investigator's colleagues and contacts. Each package included:

- Physician-to-physician referral letter, with instructions for referring a patient
- One physician-focused study brochure
- One inclusion/exclusion pocket guide
- One branded study folder

The program included packages for 100% of the sites in Canada and Germany and 50% of the sites in France, Italy, Poland and Spain. The program also included a small number of packages to accommodate any interested physicians in Czech Republic, Hungary, Greece and Tunisia. All materials were translated into the appropriate language(s) for each country.

A total of 692 physician packages were produced and distributed. Physician education packages were grossly underutilized, and funds were eventually shifted to support the production of additional recruitment kits.

Biannual Study Awareness Mailers

To maintain periodic contact between the study teams at the investigative sites and other neurologists and staff members, DAC created and provided biannual educational study awareness mailers. These allowed study coordinators an opportunity to personally distribute study information to non-study neurologists and other staff members who were interfacing with the target patient population and who could possibly refer a patient. The content included educational information (example topics included clinical research, connecting with patients, customer service in healthcare, etc.), brief trial information and instructions for referring patients. Mailers were translated into the appropriate language(s) for each country.

The program included mailers for 100% of the sites in Canada and Germany and 50% of the sites in France, Italy, Poland and Spain. The program also included a small number of mailers to accommodate interested sites in Czech Republic, Hungary, Greece and Tunisia.

Bimonthly Electronic Study Newsletters

An indirect recruitment strategy included in this program was the study newsletter. The content was drafted primarily by the sponsor, and DAC designed the newsletter using the approved messaging for the trial. Typically, the newsletter was four pages, including CRF completion tips, protocol clarifications, enrollment updates and information on how to leverage the recruitment program to supplement the site's screening efforts. The newsletter was distributed electronically directly from DAC to the sites and sponsor.

Translations

Translation was completed for all countries following finalization of the English master files. Materials translated included all patient-facing materials and the physician education materials. The table below illustrates the languages that were provided, by country.

Challenges

This recruitment program faced a number of challenges, several of which became apparent as early as the proposal/bid process. Each challenge had a varying degree of impact on the execution of the program, and the associated impact measurement is noted, where appropriate. Many of these issues persisted throughout the duration of the recruitment program, and some carried into the closeout and contract reconciliation stage. The major challenges are outlined below, with additional detail provided on each.

U.S.-based Vendor for an ex-U.S. Program

During the proposal and bid process, the sponsor shared concerns from team members that a U.S.-based company would be managing a completely ex-U.S. program. The model for global project management was shared with the client and was passed on to extended members of the team. Although mentioned throughout DAC's involvement in this program, a measurable impact on the program was not observed.

Impact Measurement: Mild

Risk Share Element

In the final stages of vendor selection, the sponsor pushed hard for vendors to commit to an aggressive risk share model. This, in essence, created a "bidding war" that revolved around the risk share element of each proposal. Confident in our program and the impact it would have, DAC put 25% of the overall program value at risk, based on the ability to guarantee 90 "referred" patients. Overall, this risk share was aggressive from DAC's perspective and

Figure 1: Sharing the model for global project management

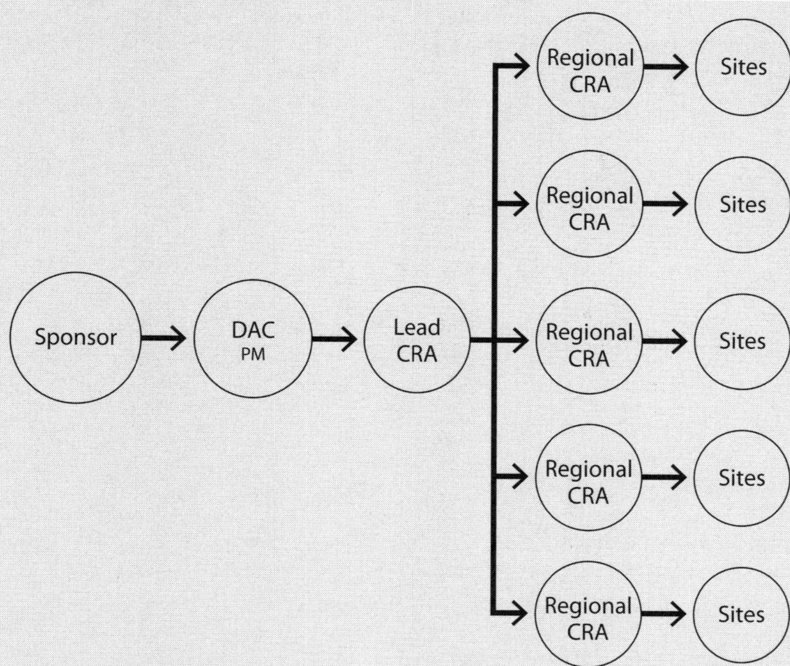

Source: DAC Patient Recruitment Services

was beyond a typical "risk" that would be associated with a program of this size.

As enrollment began, and the performance-based element of the contract became increasingly relevant, the sponsor contested the meaning of a "referred" patient. From the sponsor's perspective, value was not in the referral of a patient but in the actual randomization of a patient. The risk share was void of critical definitions that were later very difficult to negotiate, as early metrics that were available were a driving factor for both parties. Although DAC contested the "randomization" milestone, due to a number of variables (e.g., site reporting on outcomes), DAC agreed to re-define the risk share model as 90 "randomized" patients.

Impact Measurement: Mild

EC Submission/Review Timelines

There is a perception in the clinical trial industry that ethics committee timelines can be extremely lengthy. While this may be true in some countries, what should be of equal concern, and possibly greater concern, since it is a preventable delay, is the actual time to submission. Once the files were ready for submission within a given country, the files were provided to the ap-

Figure 2: File submission by country

Country	Item	Final files to local team	EC submission date	Day(s) to EC submission	Days to EC ruling
Czech	Recruitment materials	17-Jun	24-Jun	7	132
	Web site	3-Aug	19-Oct	77	15
Spain	Recruitment materials	23-Jun	2-Jul	9	53
	Web site	10-Aug	11-Aug	1	155
Italy	Recruitment materials	17-Jun	13-Jul	26	17
	Web site	5-Oct	27-Jan	114	N/A
Tunisia	Recruitment materials	18-Sep	29-Oct	41	N/A
	Web site	21-Oct	29-Oct	8	N/A
Poland	Recruitment materials	2-Jul	9-Nov	130	88
	Web site	4-Nov	9-Nov	5	88
Canada	Recruitment materials	29-Jun	N/A	N/A	N/A
	Web site	N/A	N/A	N/A	N/A
Hungary	Recruitment materials	14-Dec	13-Jan	30	84
	Web site	6-Jan	13-Jan	7	84
Germany	Recruitment materials	12-Mar	17-Mar	5	8
	Web site	N/A	N/A	N/A	N/A
France	Recruitment materials	16-Jun	22-Apr	310	46
	Web site	N/A	N/A	N/A	N/A
Belgium	Recruitment materials	25-Mar	31-Mar	6	29
	Web site	25-Mar	31-Mar	6	29
U.K.	Recruitment materials	30-Oct	20-Nov	21	76
	Web site	16-Nov	20-Nov	4	76
Switzerland	Recruitment materials	N/A	N/A	N/A	N/A

propriate team member as a zip file, with an attachment that outlined the purpose and intended target audience for each piece. DAC was available for any questions related to the materials. The table below illustrates the number of days from the date the files were submitted to the local team in each country to the date the submission was made to the EC. Additionally, the table shows the number of days from the submission to the ruling. Submission timelines exceeding three weeks are highlighted. Review timelines exceeding eight weeks are highlighted.

Impact Measurement: Severe

Matrix Sponsor Organization

The clinical trial manager was the primary point of contact for DAC. The clinical trial manager and clinical trial assistant were the consistent attendees on the DAC weekly call to review the status and progress of the program. Communication was free flowing between DAC and the internal/sponsor management team. Early in the program, it was apparent that there was a lack of responsiveness to requests placed from the clinical trial manager to the country leads and CRAs. The clinical trial manager was often unable to get a timeline response from the local teams, and the sponsor verbalized that the matrix organization was the cause. This led to a lack of accountability and responsiveness from some of the country teams. DAC worked directly with the local teams, and there was a direct correlation between the responsiveness and engagement of the team and the overall success of the program in that particular country.

Impact Measurement: Severe

Translation Feedback from Local Teams

Upon receipt of the translated files, the documents were sent electronically to the local team in each country for review and feedback. The response times varied greatly from one country to another. This created significant delays in the preparation of the EC-ready files for submission. The most likely causes of delay were a lack of engagement in the recruitment program, competing priorities by the local teams and the matrix aspect of the organization, which created a lack of accountability. The table below illustrates the number of days between the delivery of the files and receipt of feedback.

Impact Measurement: Moderate

Rigidity of Czech Translation

As noted in the table above, the feedback from the Czech Republic was received in a very short turnaround time. The translations were approved with no revisions. Upon submission of the materials to the EC in Czech Republic,

Figure 3: Translation feedback by country

Country	Item	Translation sent	Feedback received	Day(s) awaiting feedback
Czech	Recruitment materials	2-Jun	5-Jun	3
	Web site	30-Jun	1-Jul	1
Spain	Recruitment materials	2-Jun	16-Jun	14
	Web site	30-Jun	14-Jul	14
Italy	Recruitment materials	2-Jun	9-Jun	7
	Web site	30-Jun	3-Aug	34
Tunisia	Recruitment materials	14-Jul	26-Aug	43
	Web site	30-Jun	26-Aug	57
Poland	Recruitment materials	22-Jun	29-Jun	7
	Web site	30-Jun	17-Jul	17
Canada	Recruitment materials	2-Jun	15-Jun	13
	Web site	30-Jun	N/A	N/A
Hungary	Recruitment materials	2-Jun	30-Oct	150
	Web site	1-Jul	30-Oct	121
Germany	Recruitment materials	2-Jun	8-Mar	279
	Web site	30-Jun	8-Mar	251
France	Recruitment materials	2-Jun	8-Jun	6
	Web site	30-Jun	N/A	N/A
Belgium	Recruitment materials	1-Feb	24-Feb	23
	Web site	2-Feb	24-Feb	22
U.K.	Recruitment materials	22-Sep	6-Oct	14
	Web site	22-Sep	6-Oct	14
Switzerland	Recruitment materials	8-Mar	4-May	57

the local team received feedback from the EC that the rigidity of the web site translation was unacceptable. The recruitment materials were approved; however, review of the web site was tabled until an improved translation was provided. The sponsor elected to have a local translation company provide a new translation. In order to follow up on the matter and understand the issues with translation, DAC had the original translation provider perform back translation and then conducted an in-house comparison of the language. Several errors were found in the original translation, and these were shared with the sponsor. The team in Czech Republic elected not to submit the new web site language to the EC, and the web site was never launched in Czech Republic. Working through the details of this issue, the Czech team later indicated that a local review was never completed, as competing priorities did not allow the team to devote time to this.

Impact Measurement: Moderate

Risk Share Definitions

Initial risk share included milestones around "referred" patients; however, the sponsor felt that this was inadvertently misnamed and should have been "randomized" patients. After discussions between DAC and the sponsor, the risk share element was revised to allow evaluation of the milestone of randomization. Although this language intensified the commitment, it did provide a measurable milestone without the ambiguity that existed with the "referred" patient milestone.

Another challenge related to the risk share was the lack of definition around the strategies that would "count" toward the accrual of patients that would be credited to DAC's program. For example, the sponsor's position was that patient-directed recruitment materials such as the brochures, fliers, posters (i.e., the recruitment kit) should not be able to generate a randomized patient for risk share purposes, due to the fact that any patients who would see those materials were already known to the investigative sites and were therefore not "found" by DAC. This was most problematic, because the value of the risk share, in dollars, was based on 25% of the entire program value, rather than 25% of those strategies that would identify patients not currently known to the sites. A more extreme example, which further illustrates this challenge, is the bimonthly study newsletter. Although it is impossible to draw a correlation between a study newsletter and a randomized patient, the value of that service was tied into the risk share value. This was an oversight on the part of DAC, but proved to be a valuable lesson learned.

Impact Measurement: Mild

IVRS

In order to assess the impact of the recruitment program on overall screening and randomization, prompts were incorporated into the IVRS programming

Figure 4: Impact measured by IVRS

How did the patient first find out about this study?

	Subjects screened							Subjects randomized						
	IVRS prompts							IVRS prompts						
Country	**1**	**2**	**3**	**4**	**5**	**6**	**7**	**1**	**2**	**3**	**4**	**5**	**6**	**7**
Belgium	3	0	0	0	8	0	0	3	0	0	0	7	0	0
Canada	0	0	0	0	10	12	0	0	0	0	0	10	10	0
Switzerland	0	0	0	0	1	0	0	0	0	0	0	1	0	0
Czech	0	0	0	0	22	0	0	0	0	0	0	20	0	0
Germany	7	0	0	2	51	0	0	6	0	0	2	45	0	0
Spain	2	0	0	0	22	0	0	2	0	0	0	20	0	0
France	10	0	0	0	35	0	0	9	0	0	0	30	0	0
United	1	0	3	0	3	0	0	1	0	3	0	1	0	0
Greece	0	0	0	0	5	0	0	0	0	0	0	2	0	0
Hungary	2	0	0	0	27	0	0	2	0	0	0	27	0	0
Italy	8	0	0	0	47	0	0	7	0	0	0	42	0	0
Poland	3	0	0	0	64	1	1	3	0	0	0	54	1	1
Tunisia	2	0	0	0	0	0	0	1	0	0	0	0	0	0
Totals	**38**	**0**	**3**	**2**	**295**	**13**	**1**	**34**	**0**	**3**	**2**	**259**	**11**	**1**

- 1 = Physician referral (referral from another physician outside the investigative site/site's database of patients)
- 2 = Support group or other community outreach initiative
- 3 = Study web site
- 4 = Recruitment materials (poster, flier, brochure)
- 5 = Existing patient of site (internal patient database)
- 6 = Patient referral—patient was referred to the study by one of your practice's existing patients
- 7 = Patient referral—patient was referred to the study by another study patient who was informed through initiatives of the recruitment vendor, DAC

Note: Prompts 1–4, and 7 were tracked for the purpose of risk share evaluation.

for the official screening visit. DAC and the sponsor determined which of the services would be evaluated by the sites as possible primary exposure sources for screened and randomized patients. The challenge with the IVRS prompts ties into those mentioned with the risk share definitions. It was not possible to draw a direct correlation between many of the services and a screened patient. The question and prompts in Figure 4 are those that were programmed into IVRS and presented to sites.

Impact Measurement: Moderate

Incorrect Use of Prompts

Despite education of the sites and CRAs at every possible opportunity, a lack of understanding of the prompts persisted throughout the enrollment period. This was evidenced by the indication that erroneous prompts were selected for sites that did not have the corresponding strategy active. For example, the web site was indicated as a patient source in a country in which the study web site was not active. Of the screened and randomized patients attributed to DAC's program, and estimated 40% of these were erroneous.

Web Site Acceptance

Web sites are becoming a critical component of most recruitment programs, both inside and outside the U.S. There was some degree of resistance in almost all countries, and this was more easily overcome in certain countries than in others. Education and examples of previously approved web sites were used to combat the resistance. This was effective in those countries in which a web site eventually was launched.

Study Web Site in Spain

The EC in Spain does not allow collection of patient contact information. As described in the program elements section, DAC created an alternate method for generating the patient referral in the absence of a patient's contact information. Despite this alternative, it was difficult for patients to keep this number available, and it left the site with no way to reach out to patients directly. This method relied solely on the patients reaching out to the site to follow up on the pre-screening.

Outcomes and Metrics

The most important outcome related to this program is that the trial reached full accrual 2.5 months ahead of schedule.

Figure 5: Web site performance

Country	# of days web site was live	Confirmed randomized	Visitors	Pre-screened	Failed	Qualified	Actual referrals
Spain	187	-	4,285	-	-	-	68
Poland	138	-	3,760	-	-	-	73
U.K.	131	3	6,039	-	-	-	25
Belgium (Dutch/ French)	66	-	1,096	-	-	-	5
Tunisia (Arabic/ French)	89 / 54	-	577	-	-	-	1
Total	-	**3**	**15,757**	**978**	**693**	**285**	**172**

Web Site Performance

Although Spain and Poland had the highest number of referred patients, no metrics were reported from the sites related to these referrals. It is unknown how many, if any, of these patients were contacted for the study and how many may have randomized.

Overall Impact of the Recruitment Program

The overall impact on screening/randomization can be seen in the impact graph in Figure 6. The deployment of initiatives is detailed across this timeline.

Lessons Learned

The lessons learned throughout this global recruitment program have been invaluable to the success of future programs. There is an element of learn-as-you-go to almost any recruitment program, due to the rapidly changing landscape and industry regulations. Taking lessons learned and applying them to future programs brings the greatest possible benefit to a sponsor and works to shorten the recruitment timeline for trials. The following points highlight the most valuable lessons learned through the course of DAC's involvement in this recruitment program.

- Obtaining support from the local (country) teams is essential for maintaining the program timeline.

Figure 6: Program impact graph

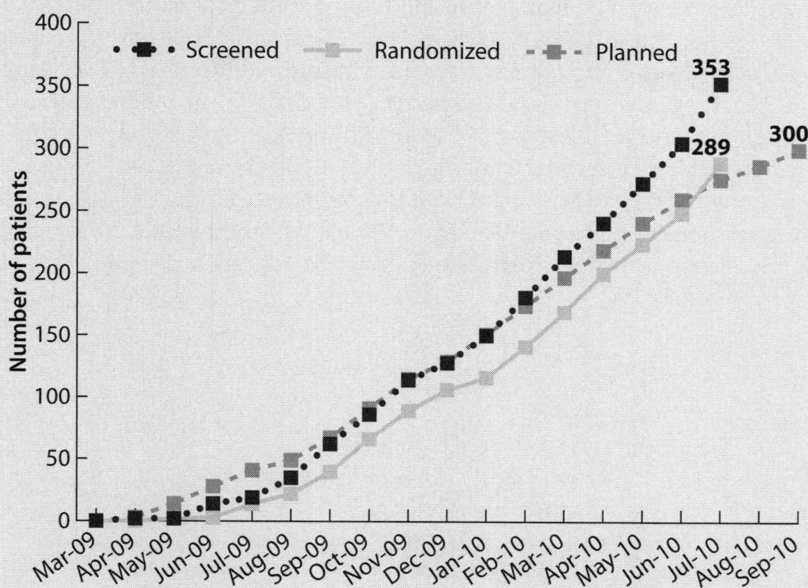

Source: DAC Patient Recruitment Services

- Risk share or performance-based pricing must be thoroughly evaluated and reviewed internally so necessary protective measures can be included prior to execution of the contract. There is a shift in a provider's ability to negotiate after contract execution.
- Risk share value should correlate to the services that can have a direct and measurable impact on recruitment
- It is perfectly reasonable (and definitely possible) to manage a recruitment program without feet on the street in participating countries. It does, however, require frequent and clear communication with key team members.
- The tracking and reporting element for sites must be strongly encouraged by the sponsor and CRAs in each country. This is a critical element in evaluating ROI.
- Never underestimate the impact a matrix organization can have on the level of accountability and responsiveness of the local teams.
- Sponsor involvement is critical in pushing translation review and timeline submission of recruitment materials to the EC.
- Physician education materials are utilized at approximately a 75% reduction ex-U.S. compared to U.S. use.

Author Biography

Lacey Powers is senior manager of medical operations at Reata Pharmaceuticals. Of her more than 10 years in the clinical trials industry, the last six have focused on global patient recruitment and retention. Prior to joining DAC, Lacey gained significant experience in the clinical research industry through her work with the U.S. Veterans' Administration, serving as a clinical research coordinator and site manager. In her current role, Lacey focuses on overseeing global patient recruitment programs and conducting training for CRCs and sponsors. Her clinical experience spans therapeutic areas including oncology, neurology, cardiology, gastroenterology, orthopedic surgery and pulmonology.

CHAPTER FOURTEEN

Close Up on Asia Pacific Rim

By Diana L. Anderson-Foster, Ph.D.

As the world's largest continent, comprising 44 countries and four billion people, Asia is replete with possibility in the clinical research realm. Recent data, available at ClinicalTrials.gov, show 5,681 trials actively recruiting participants in the North, South, Southeast and Eastern quadrants of the continent. Of particular note, a hotbed of clinical activity is underway in China—a standout economy among the BRIC (Brazil, Russia, India, and China), four countries on similarly accelerated paths of economic development.

China's double-digit annual growth rate in research and development surpasses expansion in established markets such as the United States, the United Kingdom and Japan. According to the *2010 Global R&D Funding Forecast*, China outspent Japan in R&D in 2011 and is expected to match aggressive spending in Europe in 2018 and rival U.S. R&D spending in 2022. This phenomenon is fueled by several factors, including establishment of clinical trial laws, alliance with the World Trade Organization and formation of the State Food and Drug Administration in 2003. But with progress comes new challenges, namely increased competition, cost concerns and trial delays.

Increased competition seems largely the result of continued industry consolidation—a consequence of the recent global recession, which decreased the number of biotech companies and reduced R&D funds. Further eroding industry investments are declining numbers of new products in the pipeline and increasing numbers of generic drugs. The pharmaceutical market experienced a 2 percent decline in 2009, representing the first decrease in 50 years. Current projections anticipate only a 2.2 percent annual growth rate.

Despite general downturns, the Asian markets remain resilient,offering many potential advantages from a patient recruitment perspective including access to a larger number of treatment-naive patients. A.T. Kearney, a global management consultant firm, conducted an analysis in 2009 highlighting preferred global destinations for clinical research. Among the 16 countries making the cut, five were in Asia, including number one-ranked China.

In addition to abundant patient pools, strengthening regulations and research-minded physicians, cost efficiency is a major incentive for conducting clinical trials in Asia. For example, according to some estimates, per-patient

Figure 1: BRIC in brief

Brazil

Touted as the gateway to Latin America, Brazil's strength as a clinical research center lies in numbers: a large treatment-naïve population of 201 million people, 8000 hospitals, 96 medical schools and 415 institutional review boards. While those figures are impressive for a developing country, perhaps the most important calculation is Brazil's pharmaceutical market index—a 14.5% compound annual growth rate forecast through 2014. The country has rather sophisticated guidelines governing the conduct of clinical trials, as detailed in "Rules on Research on Human Subjects" (Resolution CNS 196/96—"Normas Para Pesquisa Envolvendo Seres Humanos").

Russia

Russian study volunteers are generally very compliant in terms of keeping appointments, taking study meds and recording in patient diaries, and they rarely withdraw consent. They also seem to be highly motivated to participate in studies to gain access to the best facilities and the best physicians at no cost. Their high level of compliance may be because doctors in Russia continue to be seen as influential authority figures and patients value their opinions. Some research suggests that, on average, study subjects tend to be fairly well educated.

India

India was formerly overlooked by pharma companies because of limited intellectual property protection and the preponderance of generic pharmaceuticals produced by indigenous companies. Trial ethics also came into question following a survey by the former U.S. National Bioethics Advisory Commission that revealed 25% of clinical trials conducted in developing countries did not undergo ethical review. Today, patent protection is no longer a barrier, as India now complies with Trade-Related Aspects of Intellectual Property Rights. Additionally, the Academy for Clinical Excellence and Institute of Clinical Research have been established to educate doctors in ICH-GCP guidelines and ethical trial requirements.

China

Clinical research in China is very much an emerging enterprise. With a population of 1.3 billion, much of it treatment-naïve, the country is a highly anticipated venue for clinical trials.

Source: DAC Patient Recruitment Services

costs for clinical trials in India are approximately 40 percent to 60 percent of those in North America and Europe.

Asia's clinical potential was just capturing international attention four years ago when the author led a delegation of 10 clinical research profession-

Figure 2: China's clinical trial laws and regulations

- Drug Administration Law of the People's Republic of China—effective Dec. 1, 2001
- Regulations for Implementation of the Drug Administration of the People's Republic of China – effective Sept. 15, 2002
- Regulations for the Supervision and Administration of Medical Devices—effective April 1, 2000
- Chinese GCP Guidelines updated, 2003

Source: DAC Patient Recruitment Services

als to China to forge relations and exchange ideas for advancing the clinical trials industry. The visit was part of the Ambassador program based in Washington, D.C., and founded by former U.S. President Dwight D. Eisenhower. Its mission is to help individuals gain a better understanding of global cultures through first-hand travel experiences. Over the course of 13 days, the delegation toured four cities and met with pharmaceutical companies, hospitals, site management organizations, a pharmaceutical manufacturing plant and a contract research organization. Interactions included in-depth discussions about good clinical practice, informed consent and patient recruitment techniques.

What the group learned, and what remains true today, is that developing tactics to overcome clinical trial challenges is insufficient; you also need a comprehensive strategy for applying them. To that end, in September 2011 a two-day training session on "Effective Clinical Site Management & Patient Recruitment" in Singapore was held. This focused on understanding the importance of good site selection to assist in the navigation of the clinical trial process, developing a strong working relationship to ensure proper conduct of the trial in accordance with applicable laws and regulations, building and maintaining a successful budget through contract and finance monitoring, achieving an international standard multi-centered clinical site and designing an advanced patient recruitment and retention plan for a seamless trial.

A DAC survey of 25 session attendees, all of whom work and reside in Asia, revealed that while the region has many positive attributes for conducting clinical trials, lack of awareness, coupled with trial delays, hinder the process. Attendees identified ethics committee approval times, competing studies and investigator selection as reasons for delays. Reported EC approval times ranged widely from two weeks to three months, but perhaps the most significant delays occur before enrollment even gets underway. In China it can take nine to 12 months to obtain approval from the State Food and Drug Administration (SFDA) to conduct a trial. Add to that the time required to evaluate and initiate sites, obtain drug import licenses and recruit patients, and the delays can seem insurmountable.

Figure 3: Overall country attractiveness index

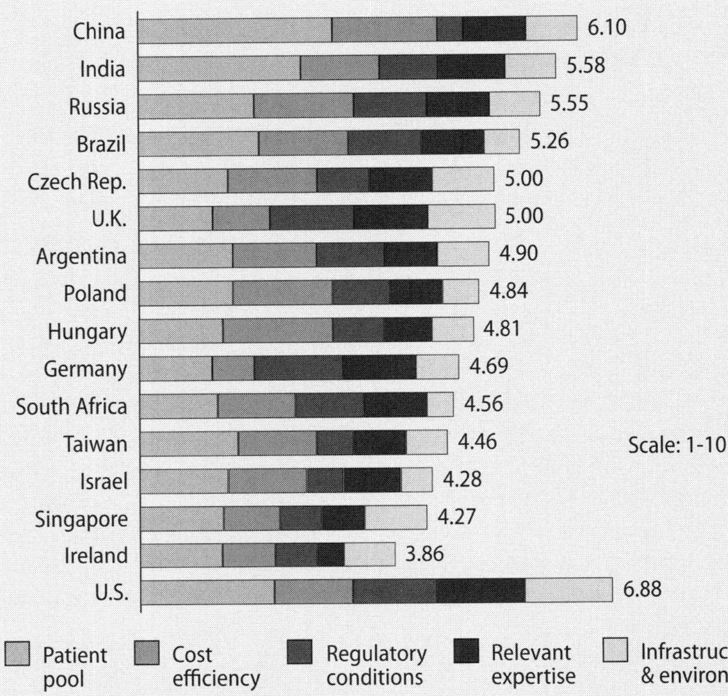

Note: The 15 countries analyzed were selected based on size, diversity and geographical distribution. The index is not meant to be comprehensive across all potential offshore locations.

Source: A.T. Kearney, 2009

Variances in Recruitment Regulations

The regulatory and ethical climates relating to recruitment practices differ regionally and dissecting the guidelines can be difficult. The need for recruitment support in Asia depends on how recruitment is defined. When viewed from the standpoint of strict direct-to-patient study awareness strategies, external patient recruitment initiatives may be less relevant or appropriate in densely populated areas with specialized healthcare institutions than in other areas where patient access is more restrictive due to geographic spread or competing trials. For these regions, tools and materials developed to facilitate patient identification within individual institutions are more appropriate than public awareness-building campaigns.

Based on extensive research and practical experience supporting patient recruitment in 100 countries, DAC has found that patient recruitment is rarely mentioned in government regulations. When included, most of the guidelines discuss recruitment methods in the context of requiring ethics committee review but rarely explicitly address whether certain strategies are

Figure 4: Enrollment delays

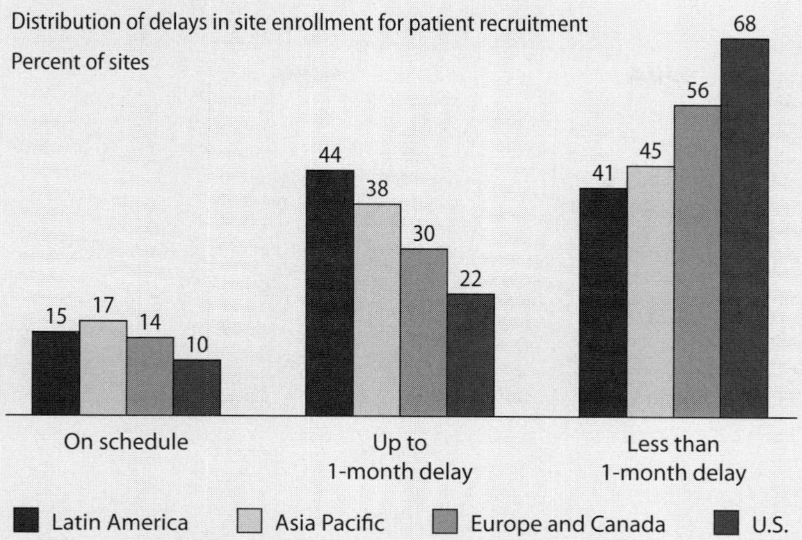

Source: CenterWatch surveys of U.S. (2009, n=950), Asian (2006, n=156), Latin American (2005, n=317), European and Canadian (2006, n=356) investigative sites

allowed or prohibited. For many countries, recruitment methods are deemed permissible as long as an ethics committee approves the proposed methods. Many recruitment strategies commonly used in the U.S. are seldom employed globally, based more on tradition than on regulatory restrictions. Regulations will broaden to support activities as more clinical trials are conducted in Asia. As regulations are refined and geographical borders blend, the region is awakening to traditional Western methods of reaching subjects, including call centers, web site marketing and social networking, among other tools.

Recruitment strategies and challenges aside, another confounding aspect of clinical trial management in Asian culture is patient retention, according to Theshinee Chuenyan, R.N., head of clinical and office operations at IATEC—a CRO based in Bangkok, Thailand. Chuenyan suggests the paternalistic relationship between patients and doctors facilitates compliance with trial participation, whereas inadequate follow-up contributes to attrition.

"Getting patients to participate in a clinical trial is not as much of a problem because it is customary in Asian culture for patients to comply with their doctor's requests," she said. "Not enough emphasis is placed on informed consent; therefore, patients are inadequately educated about the process of clinical trial participation. Also lacking are educational materials and communication to keep patients engaged until the trial ends. Over time they simply drop out."

DAC's survey respondents echoed these sentiments, noting patients' general lack of awareness about their rights and underscoring the importance of

Figure 5: Regulatory environment for Asia Pacific

Country	Current SSV-SIV times (Avg days)	Comments
Singapore	203	Amended insurance coverage regulations
Malaysia	217	1. Products of bovine/porcine origin to be listed ICF as well as labels 2. Imports from Israel banned
Philippines	200	New requirement for withholding tax delaying CTA execution
Taiwan	270	Challenging CTA negotiations—Q template heavily recommended
Korea	215	Lab kit import license now required
Thailand	210	MOPH site taking longer for EC approval
Vietnam	245	
Indonesia	267	Review on export of biological samples expected soon
Hong Kong	206	Drug sample (dummy) required for RA submission
India	265	License required from DGFT to export blood samples (+2 weeks)

Source: DAC Patient Recruitment Services

the doctor-patient relationship in averting attrition.

Using strategies reminiscent of the now-obsolete Western tradition of "making house calls," Chuenyan and her colleagues maintained less than 5 percent attrition in an HIV clinical research trial in Cambodia by dispatching nurses to villages to check on study participants, answer questions and provide personalized care. While such tactics are likely time- and cost-prohibitive for most clinicians, they should serve as a guide for going the full distance to retain trial participants.

Developing effective and informative patient education materials is a must in the clinical trials industry. Nowhere is this more important than in the informed consent document. One of the primary principles regarding informed consent is that "the information that is given to the subject or the representative shall be in language understandable to the subject or the representative."[1] Due to the highly technical nature of investigational research, presenting complex information in the simplest form can be challenging.

In general, health-related information is more difficult to comprehend than most other types of information. In the U.S., per Food and Drug Administration (FDA) regulations, institutional review boards (IRBs) ensure that technical and scientific terms are adequately explained and that the informed consent document properly translates complex concepts into simple language that the "typical" subject can read and comprehend. Most IRBs stipulate reading levels for such documents as part of their responsibility to ensure that research subjects understand the informed consent. Similarly, ethics committees may require that the consent form be written below a specific grade level to more appropriately reflect the reading levels within the community from which prospective subjects will be recruited. While regulations directly address requirements for the informed consent document, these principles apply to any type of patient educational materials.

Written informed consent forms are gradually being promoted and implemented in Asia to meet the requirements of good clinical practice (GCP). Prior to the issue of GCP in 1999, many people were unfamiliar with the clinical trial as an emerging area. Asian people conventionally regarded the signature as something similar to a self-selling indenture. As a result, many subjects still orally agree to cooperate in trials but refuse to sign their names on the written document.

To mitigate these issues, measures are being taken in Asia to protect trial subjects, including establishing GCP training centers for clinical trial investigators, doctors, pharmacists and sponsors; setting up a system to periodically evaluate clinical trial bases; and legally protecting subjects' benefits and rights.

Such progress is encouraging. Despite the preponderance of treatment-naïve patients and other attributes, clinicians in Asia are under no illusion that meeting enrollment goals is a sure thing. There remains a high unmet need for targeted patient recruitment and retention strategies, as well as continued education on ethics and law. Astuteness in regulatory requirements is but one prerequisite for implementing an effective recruitment and retention program in Asia. A number of variables contribute to success, including the establishment of rapport, trust and mutual commitment to study goals among research sites, the CRO and the sponsor. From these relationships arises enthusiasm among sites to embrace and execute recruitment strategies.

Taking the time to invest in relationships may be the best recruitment strategy of all. Beyond their oversight, institutional policies and physician attitudes can heavily influence recruitment and retention practices. The lines of communication must remain open to ensure strategies are understood and fully executed. In doing so, sites will be better equipped to manage challenges as they arise and employ methods to avoid study delays.

Figure 6: Asia Pacific recruitment strategies: China

Recruitment strategies	Acceptable per regs	Average use by sites	Recommended by DAC
Patient education materials (brochures, fliers, posters, etc.)	Yes	50-75%	Yes
Study awareness and patient identification toolkits for sites	Yes	100%	Yes
Physician-to-patient letters/ study awareness packets	Yes	50-75%	Yes
Physician education packages and follow-up mailers (medical community outreach)	Yes	50%	Yes
Physician outreach/education events (dinners and web presentations)	Yes	0-25%	CC
Physician community/advocacy group outreach (direct-to-patient)	Yes	50%	Yes
Study web site	NP	ND	CC
Web marketing (pay-per-click, AdWords and banner advertising)	NP	ND	CC
Direct-to-patient advertising (print, radio & TV)	NP	ND	CC
Patient e-messaging	ND	ND	No
Retention strategies			
Call center	Yes	ND	No
Patient education materials (brochures, booklets, newsletters, etc.)	Yes	50-100%	Yes
Patient compliance items (custom calendars, study diaries, etc.)	Yes	50-100%	Yes
Patient retention text and e-messaging	NP	ND	Yes
Transportation assistance program/ClinCard debit cards	NP	ND	CC

CC: Case-by-case basis ND: No data NP: Not specifically prohibited by regs

Source: DAC Patient Recruitment Services

Figure 7: Asia Pacific recruitment strategies: Hong Kong

Recruitment strategies	Acceptable per regs	Average use by sites	Recommended by DAC
Patient education materials (brochures, fliers, posters, etc.)	Yes	50-75%	Yes
Study awareness and patient identification toolkits for sites	Yes	100%	Yes
Physician-to-patient letters/ study awareness packets	Yes	50-75%	Yes
Physician education packages and follow-up mailers (medical community outreach)	Yes	50%	Yes
Physician outreach/education events (dinners and web presentations)	Yes	0-25%	CC
Physician community/advocacy group outreach (direct-to-patient)	Yes	50%	Yes
Study web site	NP	ND	CC
Web marketing (pay-per-click, AdWords and banner advertising)	NP	ND	CC
Direct-to-patient advertising (print, radio & TV)	ND	ND	CC
Patient e-messaging	ND	ND	No
Retention strategies			
Call center	Yes	ND	No
Patient education materials (brochures, booklets, newsletters, etc.)	Yes	50-100%	Yes
Patient compliance items (custom calendars, study diaries, etc.)	Yes	50-100%	Yes
Patient retention text and e-messaging	NP	ND	Yes
Transportation assistance program/ClinCard debit cards	ND	ND	CC

CC: Case-by-case basis ND: No data NP: Not specifically prohibited by regs

Source: DAC Patient Recruitment Services

Figure 8: Asia Pacific recruitment strategies: Indonesia

Recruitment strategies	Acceptable per regs	Average use by sites	Recommended by DAC
Patient education materials (brochures, fliers, posters, etc.)	Yes	50-75%	Yes
Study awareness and patient identification toolkits for sites	Yes	100%	Yes
Physician-to-patient letters/ study awareness packets	Yes	50-75%	Yes
Physician education packages and follow-up mailers (medical community outreach)	Yes	50%	Yes
Physician outreach/education events (dinners and web presentations)	Yes	0-25%	CC
Physician community/advocacy group outreach (direct-to-patient)	Yes	50%	Yes
Study web site	ND	ND	CC
Web marketing (pay-per-click, AdWords and banner advertising)	ND	ND	CC
Direct-to-patient advertising (print, radio & TV)	ND	ND	CC
Patient e-messaging	ND	ND	No
Retention strategies			
Call center	Yes	ND	No
Patient education materials (brochures, booklets, newsletters, etc.)	Yes	50-100%	Yes
Patient compliance items (custom calendars, study diaries, etc.)	Yes	50-100%	Yes
Patient retention text and e-messaging	NP	ND	Yes
Transportation assistance program/ClinCard debit cards	ND	ND	CC

CC: Case-by-case basis ND: No data NP: Not specifically prohibited by regs

Source: DAC Patient Recruitment Services

Figure 9: Asia Pacific recruitment strategies: India

Recruitment strategies	Acceptable per regs	Average use by sites	Recommended by DAC
Patient education materials (brochures, fliers, posters, etc.)	Yes	50-75%	Yes
Study awareness and patient identification toolkits for sites	Yes	100%	Yes
Physician-to-patient letters/ study awareness packets	Yes	50-75%	Yes
Physician education packages and follow-up mailers (medical community outreach)	Yes	50%	Yes
Physician outreach/education events (dinners and web presentations)	Yes	0-25%	CC
Physician community/advocacy group outreach (direct-to-patient)	Yes	50%	Yes
Study web site	Yes	50%	Yes
Web marketing (pay-per-click, AdWords and banner advertising)	Yes	50%	Yes
Direct-to-patient advertising (print, radio & TV)	NP	ND	CC
Patient e-messaging	ND	ND	No
Retention strategies			
Call center	Yes	ND	No
Patient education materials (brochures, booklets, newsletters, etc.)	Yes	50-100%	Yes
Patient compliance items (custom calendars, study diaries, etc.)	Yes	50-100%	Yes
Patient retention text and e-messaging	NP	ND	Yes
Transportation assistance program/ClinCard debit cards	NP	ND	CC

CC: Case-by-case basis ND: No data NP: Not specifically prohibited by regs

Source: DAC Patient Recruitment Services

Figure 10: Asia Pacific recruitment strategies: Japan

Recruitment strategies	Acceptable per regs	Average use by sites	Recommended by DAC
Patient education materials (brochures, fliers, posters, etc.)	Yes	75-100%	Yes
Study awareness and patient identification toolkits for sites	Yes	100%	Yes
Physician-to-patient letters/ study awareness packets	Yes	75-100%	Yes
Physician education packages and follow-up mailers (medical community outreach)	Yes	50%	Yes
Physician outreach/education events (dinners and web presentations)	Yes	0-25%	CC
Physician community/advocacy group outreach (direct-to-patient)	Yes	50%	Yes
Study web site	ND	ND	CC
Web marketing (pay-per-click, AdWords and banner advertising)	ND	ND	CC
Direct-to-patient advertising (print, radio & TV)	NP	ND	CC
Patient e-messaging	ND	ND	No
Retention strategies			
Call center	Yes	ND	No
Patient education materials (brochures, booklets, newsletters, etc.)	Yes	50-100%	Yes
Patient compliance items (custom calendars, study diaries, etc.)	Yes	50-100%	Yes
Patient retention text and e-messaging	NP	ND	Yes
Transportation assistance program/ClinCard debit cards	ND	ND	CC

CC: Case-by-case basis ND: No data NP: Not specifically prohibited by regs

Source: DAC Patient Recruitment Services

Figure 11: Asia Pacific recruitment strategies: Korea

Recruitment strategies	Acceptable per regs	Average use by sites	Recommended by DAC
Patient education materials (brochures, fliers, posters, etc.)	Yes	50-75%	Yes
Study awareness and patient identification toolkits for sites	Yes	100%	Yes
Physician-to-patient letters/ study awareness packets	Yes	50-75%	Yes
Physician education packages and follow-up mailers (medical community outreach)	Yes	50%	Yes
Physician outreach/education events (dinners and web presentations)	Yes	0-25%	CC
Physician community/advocacy group outreach (direct-to-patient)	Yes	50%	Yes
Study web site	NP	ND	CC
Web marketing (pay-per-click, AdWords and banner advertising)	NP	ND	CC
Direct-to-patient advertising (print, radio & TV)	ND	ND	CC
Patient e-messaging	ND	ND	No
Retention strategies			
Call center	Yes	ND	No
Patient education materials (brochures, booklets, newsletters, etc.)	Yes	50-100%	Yes
Patient compliance items (custom calendars, study diaries, etc.)	Yes	50-100%	Yes
Patient retention text and e-messaging	NP	ND	Yes
Transportation assistance program/ClinCard debit cards	NP	75-100%	CC

CC: Case-by-case basis ND: No data NP: Not specifically prohibited by regs

Source: DAC Patient Recruitment Services

Figure 12: Asia Pacific recruitment strategies: Malaysia

Recruitment strategies	Acceptable per regs	Average use by sites	Recommended by DAC
Patient education materials (brochures, fliers, posters, etc.)	Yes	50%	Yes
Study awareness and patient identification toolkits for sites	Yes	100%	Yes
Physician-to-patient letters/ study awareness packets	Yes	50%	Yes
Physician education packages and follow-up mailers (medical community outreach)	Yes	50%	Yes
Physician outreach/education events (dinners and web presentations)	Yes	0-25%	CC
Physician community/advocacy group outreach (direct-to-patient)	Yes	50%	Yes
Study web site	ND	ND	CC
Web marketing (pay-per-click, AdWords and banner advertising)	ND	ND	CC
Direct-to-patient advertising (print, radio & TV)	ND	ND	CC
Patient e-messaging	ND	ND	No
Retention strategies			
Call center	Yes	ND	No
Patient education materials (brochures, booklets, newsletters, etc.)	Yes	50-100%	Yes
Patient compliance items (custom calendars, study diaries, etc.)	Yes	50-100%	Yes
Patient retention text and e-messaging	NP	ND	Yes
Transportation assistance program/ClinCard debit cards	ND	ND	CC

CC: Case-by-case basis ND: No data NP: Not specifically prohibited by regs

Source: DAC Patient Recruitment Services

Figure 13: Asia Pacific recruitment strategies: Philippines

Recruitment strategies	Acceptable per regs	Average use by sites	Recommended by DAC
Patient education materials (brochures, fliers, posters, etc.)	Yes	50-75%	Yes
Study awareness and patient identification toolkits for sites	Yes	100%	Yes
Physician-to-patient letters/ study awareness packets	Yes	50-75%	Yes
Physician education packages and follow-up mailers (medical community outreach)	Yes	50%	Yes
Physician outreach/education events (dinners and web presentations)	Yes	0-25%	CC
Physician community/advocacy group outreach (direct-to-patient)	Yes	50%	Yes
Study web site	ND	ND	CC
Web marketing (pay-per-click, AdWords and banner advertising)	ND	ND	CC
Direct-to-patient advertising (print, radio & TV)	ND	ND	CC
Patient e-messaging	ND	ND	No
Retention strategies			
Call center	Yes	ND	No
Patient education materials (brochures, booklets, newsletters, etc.)	Yes	50-100%	Yes
Patient compliance items (custom calendars, study diaries, etc.)	Yes	50-100%	Yes
Patient retention text and e-messaging	NP	ND	Yes
Transportation assistance program/ClinCard debit cards	ND	75-100%	CC

CC: Case-by-case basis ND: No data NP: Not specifically prohibited by regs

Source: DAC Patient Recruitment Services

Figure 14: Asia Pacific recruitment strategies: Singapore

Recruitment strategies	Acceptable per regs	Average use by sites	Recommended by DAC
Patient education materials (brochures, fliers, posters, etc.)	Yes	50-75%	Yes
Study awareness and patient identification toolkits for sites	Yes	100%	Yes
Physician-to-patient letters/ study awareness packets	Yes	50-75%	Yes
Physician education packages and follow-up mailers (medical community outreach)	Yes	50%	Yes
Physician outreach/education events (dinners and web presentations)	Yes	0-25%	CC
Physician community/advocacy group outreach (direct-to-patient)	Yes	50%	Yes
Study web site	ND	ND	CC
Web marketing (pay-per-click, AdWords and banner advertising)	ND	ND	CC
Direct-to-patient advertising (print, radio & TV)	ND	ND	CC
Patient e-messaging	ND	ND	No
Retention strategies			
Call center	Yes	ND	No
Patient education materials (brochures, booklets, newsletters, etc.)	Yes	50-100%	Yes
Patient compliance items (custom calendars, study diaries, etc.)	Yes	50-100%	Yes
Patient retention text and e-messaging	NP	ND	Yes
Transportation assistance program/ClinCard debit cards	ND	75-100%	CC

CC: Case-by-case basis ND: No data NP: Not specifically prohibited by regs

Source: DAC Patient Recruitment Services

Figure 15: Asia Pacific recruitment strategies: Taiwan

Recruitment strategies	Acceptable per regs	Average use by sites	Recommended by DAC
Patient education materials (brochures, fliers, posters, etc.)	Yes	50-75%	Yes
Study awareness and patient identification toolkits for sites	Yes	100%	Yes
Physician-to-patient letters/ study awareness packets	Yes	50-75%	Yes
Physician education packages and follow-up mailers (medical community outreach)	Yes	50%	Yes
Physician outreach/education events (dinners and web presentations)	Yes	0-25%	CC
Physician community/advocacy group outreach (direct-to-patient)	Yes	50%	Yes
Study web site	NP	ND	CC
Web marketing (pay-per-click, AdWords and banner advertising)	NP	ND	CC
Direct-to-patient advertising (print, radio & TV)	NP	ND	CC
Patient e-messaging	ND	ND	No
Retention strategies			
Call center	Yes	ND	No
Patient education materials (brochures, booklets, newsletters, etc.)	Yes	50-100%	Yes
Patient compliance items (custom calendars, study diaries, etc.)	Yes	50-100%	Yes
Patient retention text and e-messaging	NP	ND	Yes
Transportation assistance program/ClinCard debit cards	NP	75-100%	CC

CC: Case-by-case basis ND: No data NP: Not specifically prohibited by regs

Source: DAC Patient Recruitment Services

Figure 16: Asia Pacific recruitment strategies: Thailand

Recruitment strategies	Acceptable per regs	Average use by sites	Recommended by DAC
Patient education materials (brochures, fliers, posters, etc.)	Yes	50-75%	Yes
Study awareness and patient identification toolkits for sites	Yes	100%	Yes
Physician-to-patient letters/ study awareness packets	Yes	50-75%	Yes
Physician education packages and follow-up mailers (medical community outreach)	Yes	50%	Yes
Physician outreach/education events (dinners and web presentations)	Yes	0-25%	CC
Physician community/advocacy group outreach (direct-to-patient)	Yes	50%	Yes
Study web site	ND	ND	CC
Web marketing (pay-per-click, AdWords and banner advertising)	ND	ND	CC
Direct-to-patient advertising (print, radio & TV)	ND	ND	CC
Patient e-messaging	ND	ND	No
Retention strategies			
Call center	Yes	ND	No
Patient education materials (brochures, booklets, newsletters, etc.)	Yes	50-100%	Yes
Patient compliance items (custom calendars, study diaries, etc.)	Yes	50-100%	Yes
Patient retention text and e-messaging	NP	ND	Yes
Transportation assistance program/ClinCard debit cards	ND	ND	CC

CC: Case-by-case basis ND: No data NP: Not specifically prohibited by regs

Source: DAC Patient Recruitment Services

Author Biography

Over a career spanning more than 25 years, Diana L. Anderson-Foster, Ph.D., has helped pioneer best practices in patient recruitment and retention for global clinical trials—first as founder, president and CEO of D. Anderson & Company and today as president of DAC Patient Recruitment Services, an Imperial company. Her book credits include *International Patient Recruitment: Regulatory Guidelines, Customs and Practices*; *A Guide to Patient Recruitment*; and *A Guide to Patient Recruitment and Retention*. In 2006, *PharmaVOICE* named her among the 100 Most Inspiring People in the Life Sciences Industry. She also received an International Women of Influence Award from the Global EXEC Women's International Council in 2008, among other honors.

References

1. 21 CFR 50.20 – General Requirements for Informed Consent.

CHAPTER FIFTEEN

Close Up on Eastern and Western Europe

By Diana L. Anderson-Foster, Ph.D.

As companies seek to curb the increasingly high cost of conducting clinical trials, Europe's market profile has risen, largely due to comparatively low costs, centralized medical systems and high numbers of treatment-naïve patients in densely populated communities from Iceland to the Ural Mountains. The collapse of the Soviet Union and dissolution of geopolitical lines dividing East and West have yielded integration of European Medicines Agency (EMA) regulations governing clinical trials among European Union, non-European Union and Commonwealth of Independent States members. As a result, the number of biotechnology companies in Europe has multiplied ten-fold during the past decade, with thousands today collectively shedding light on cell biology and pioneering medicinal products to address the disease burden arising from Europe's aging population. (See sidebar)

According to Insight Pharma Reports, 2.5% of global clinical trials were being conducted in Bulgaria, Cyprus, Czech Republic, Estonia, Hungary, Latvia, Lithuania, Poland, Romania, Slovakia and Slovenia as recently as 2007.[1] What's more, retention rates in the region, namely Eastern Europe, rival other areas, with 75% of subjects retained through study completion in the United States and Western Europe compared to 80% to 90% in Eastern Europe.[2]

Reports from the European Federation of Pharmaceutical Industry Associations (EFPIA), a Brussels-based trade union representing the research-based pharmaceutical industry in Europe, indicate that pharmaceutical research and development represents 17% of E.U. business investments and approximately 3.5% of total E.U. manufacturing. Of particular note, Europe is the center of vaccine research and manufacturing, accounting for about 90.2% of global production.

It takes an average 10 to 13 years and up to €700 million (approximately $922.3 million) to bring one investigational product to market in Europe. Only one drug candidate in 5,000 will become a marketable medicine. Facilitating and accelerating drug development is the philosophy behind the Innovative Medicines Initiative (IMI), a private-public partnership between the European Commission and the EFPIA. Its aim is to conduct research and to develop new and better methods for predicting the safety and efficacy of investigational drugs. With a total budget of €2 billion (approximately $2.64 billion) through 2013, IMI's therapeutic focal points are cancer, central nervous system disorders and inflammatory, metabolic and infectious diseases.

Dubious Distinction

Global accounting firm Ernst & Young reports steady growth in the phase II pipeline of European biotechs over the past five years. However, growth in the phase III pipeline and product approvals was comparatively low. E&Y's *Beyond Borders: Global Biotechnology Report 2011* states: "A significant portion of the industry's capital resources is focused on achieving proof-of-concept data to license the products to larger players or to enable a merger-and-acquisition (M&A) exit."[3]

In the days preceding the EFPIA's June 14, 2011 annual meeting in Brussels, Director-General Richard Bergström was quoted as saying, "Break-

Figure 1: European clinical pipeline by country, 2010

While certain countries showed impressive gains in their pipelines (such as Austria's 31% increase and Spain's 17% increase), the majority of countries maintained their 2009 positions.

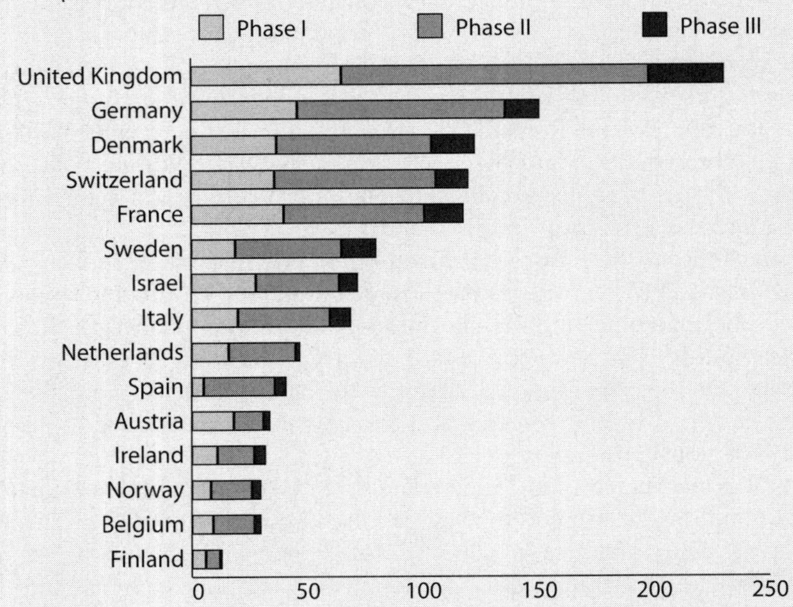

Source: Ernst & Young, MedTRACK and company web sites

through innovation in the way we understand biology and how the human body works has resulted in a bigger pipeline of medicines than ever before. Yet, there are significant challenges in delivering these to patients and in an equitable way."

Economic Setbacks

Just as the economy began to stir from a decade of stagnation that shook the region's self-confidence, Europe again is facing a recession that threatens the future of pharmaceutical R&D.

"The outlook for the European economy has deteriorated," said E.U. Economic and Monetary Affairs Commissioner Olli Rehn during the European Commission's Sept. 15, 2011 interim forecast. "Recoveries from financial crises are often slow and bumpy. Moreover, the E.U. economy is affected by a more difficult external environment, while domestic demand remains subdued. The sovereign debt crisis has worsened, and the financial market turmoil is set to dampen the real economy."

Within the pharmaceutical industry, formidable challenges exist as summarized below in a 2010 report by the EFPIA.[4]

- The costs of pharmaceutical R&D have soared due to a variety of factors including the increasingly complex nature of science and the size of clinical trials, which require more participants than ever. The latest study estimated the average cost of researching and developing a new chemical or biological entity at €1.06 billion (approximately $1.40 billion).

- There is rapid growth in the market and research environment in other emerging economies such as Brazil, China and India, resulting in further migration of economic and research activities outside Europe. According to the March 2010 IMS Health forecasts, emerging economies' pharmaceutical markets are expected to grow at a 14% to 17% rate through 2014.

- Innovation uptake remains slow in most European markets. According to data from IMS Health, 61% of sales of new medicines launched during the period from 2005 to 2009 were on the U.S. market, compared with 29% on the European market. In 2009, North America accounted for 39.8% of world pharmaceutical sales, compared with 30.6% for Europe.

- The fragmentation of the E.U. pharmaceutical market has resulted in lucrative parallel trade. This benefits neither social security nor patients and deprives the industry of additional resources to fund R&D. Parallel trade was estimated to amount to €4.4 billion (approximately $5.79 billion) (value at ex-factory prices) in 2008.

Figure 2: Selected approvals by European companies, 2010

Company	Brand name	Generic name	Type of approval
Adienne	TEPADINA	Thiotepa	New molecular entity
AOP Orphan Pharmaceuticals	TETMODIS	Tetrabenazine	New molecular entity
Archimedes Pharma	PecFent	Fentanyl	New molecular entity
AstraZeneca	BRILIQUE	Ticagrelor	Biologic license application
Bayer	Natazia	Estradiol valerate/ dienogest tabs	New molecular entity
BioAlliance Pharma	Setofilm	Ondansetron	New molecular entity
BioPartners	Ravanex	Ribavirin	New molecular entity
Boehringer Ingelheim	PRADAXA	Dabigatran	New molecular entity
Chemische Fabrik Kreussier	Asclera	Polidocanol	New molecular entity
HRA Pharma (licensed by Watson Pharmaceuticals)	ella	Ulipristal acetate	New molecular entity
Merz Pharmaceuticals	XEOMIN	IncobotulinumtoxinA	New molecular entity
Novartis	Gilenya	Fingolimod	New molecular entity
Novo Nordisk	Victoza	Liraglutide	New molecular entity
Nycomed (licensed by Baxter in U.S.)	TachoSil	Fibrin sealant patch	Biologic license application
Orphan Europe	Carbaglu	Carglumic acid	New molecular entity
Pharming Group	Ruconest	Conestat alfa	Biologic license application
Roche (R&D collaboration with Chugai)	ACTEMRA	Tocilizumab	Biologic license application
Sanofi	JEVTANA	Cabazitaxel	New molecular entity
Shire	VPRIV	Velaglucerase alfa IV	New molecular entity

*Previously approved in other markets

In aggregate, European countries had more new product approvals than their U.S. counterparts. other markets. A noteworthy U.S. approval was Shire's VPRIV, which was approved to treat Gauch supply constraints due to manufacturing problems.

Indication	Month	Orphan designation	Approved/registered in
Hematopoietic stem cell transplantation	March	Yes	E.U.
Huntington's disease	August		E.U.
Pain associated with cancer	August		E.U.
Acute coronary syndrome	December		E.U.
Pregnancy prevention	May		U.S.
Nausea and vomiting	March		16 European countries
Hepatitis C	April		E.U.
Atrial fibrillation	October		U.S.*
Small varicose veins	March		U.S.*
Pregnancy prevention	August		U.S.*
Cervical dystonia	July		U.S.*
Multiple sclerosis	September		U.S.*
Diabetes Type 2	January		U.S.*
Wound healing	April		U.S.*
Acute hyperammonemia	February	Yes	U.S.*
Hereditary angioedema	October	Yes	E.U.
Rheumatoid arthritis	January		U.S.*
Prostate cancer	June		U.S.
Gaucher's disease	February	Yes	U.S.

ignificant number represented the U.S. approval of drugs that had previously been approved in
t a time when the only other therapy for this rare condition, Genzyme's Cerezyme, was facing

Source: Ernst & Young, EMA, FDA and company web sites

Disease burden in Europe

- Each year cardiovascular disease (CVD) causes over 4.3 million deaths in Europe and over 2.0 million deaths in the European Union. Overall CVD is estimated to cost the EU economy €192 billion a year. (Source: European Heart Network)
- Cancer in Europe affects 1 in 3 men and 1 in 4 women at some time in their lives. It is estimated that 1,2 million EU citizens die from cancer each year, amounting to one in four people. (Source: Public Health Portal of the European Union)
- Tobacco is the single-largest cause of avoidable death in the EU accounting for over 650,000 deaths each year. Sickness and death caused by smoking costs EU countries at least €100 billion a year, the equivalent of 1 percent of GDP. (Source: European Public Health Alliance)
- Some 30 to 80 percent of the adult population in the WHO European Region is overweight. Obesity affects up to a third of the adult population in the region. Almost 400 million adults in the region are estimated to be overweight and about 130 million, obese. Obesity creates a major economic burden through loss of productivity and income, and consumes 2 to 8 percent of overall healthcare budgets. (Source: World Health Organization)
- 80 million people in Europe have some form of allergic disease and their prevalence is increasing.
- Around 30 million people have asthma, and as many as 6 million suffer symptoms. The full financial impact of allergic diseases to European health systems is estimated to be around €100 billion a year. (Source: European Federation of Allergy and Airway Diseases Patients Association)
- Some 23 million people are diagnosed as having depression. But many more cases are not recognized. About 40 percent of patients with severe depression are not getting any of the treatment they need. (Source: European Alliance against Depression)
- Diabetes currently affects 246 million people worldwide and is expected to affect 380 million by 2025. Each year 3.8 million deaths are attributable to diabetes. (Source: International Diabetes Federation)
- Alzheimer's disease affects about 26 million people worldwide. With an increasing aged population, that number is expected to be four times that of today by 2050. (Source: Alzheimer Europe)
- Osteoporosis affects an estimated 75 million people in Europe, USA and Japan. The total direct costs are estimated at €31.7 billion and expected to increase to €76.7 billion in 2050 based on expected changes in the demography of Europe. (Source: International Osteoporosis Foundation)
- An estimated 7 million people will suffer from epilepsy at some time during their lives. (Source: European Concerted Action and Research in Epilepsy - EUCARE)
- Schizophrenia affects 1 in 100 people at some pointing their lives with about 1.9 million cases in Europe. (Source: World Health Organization)

Disease burden in Europe

- In 2007, 33.2 million people were estimated to be living with HIV/AIDS, 2.5 million people became newly infected and 2.1 million people died of HIV/AIDS. (Source: World Health Organization)
- Almost 1.2 million people are estimated to have Parkinson's disease, with about 75,000 new cases diagnosed every year. (Source: European Parkinson's Disease Association)

The report says the pharmaceutical research-based sector "is an important engine of economic recovery," and "continued support for innovation and R&D will help Europe to regain its global leadership in pharmaceutical R&D."

To get the recovery back on track, Rehn said, "it is crucial to safeguard financial stability and put budgets on a path that is sustainable beyond doubt. This requires steadfast continuation of the strategy of differentiated, growth-friendly fiscal consolidation and the implementation of the decisions to support financial stability. At the same time, structural reforms remain more important than ever to build tomorrow's growth potential."

Calls for Change

Within the biopharmaceutical industry, among the structural reforms on the horizon is the consolidation of requirements and processes for registering clinical trials across sovereign states. Harmonization was the original intent of the Clinical Trials Directive, adopted in 2001 and implemented in 2004 by E.U. member states. However, centralized trial registration notwithstanding, the directive has been anything but harmonious. As it stands, member states disagree on interpretation of the directive. Therefore, regulatory procedures and required documents vary from one state to another, leading to paperwork duplication, wasted resources and roadblocks to approving, insuring and recruiting patients for clinical trials.

Additionally, the EFPIA has expressed support for the release of almost all clinical data as opposed to summary results. "Now is the time to take another step toward full transparency," said Bergström in an EFPIA press release.

"There will be details on patients and individuals that need to be protected, but beyond that I think all clinical test results should be disclosed as soon as a new medicine is approved," he said. "The real challenge now is to find practical ways to make this data useful. No one will benefit from a 'data dump.' Industry and regulators must work with patient groups to make sure that data is provided in a way that is helpful for patients and relatives. New tools are needed to help users navigate and understand the vast amount of data that will be released. In particular, the concept of benefit-risk needs to

Figure 3: Recruitment strategies, average usage by sites

	Austria	Belgium	Czech	Hungary	Russia	Slovakia	Ukraina
Patient education materials	50-75%	50-75%	50-75%	50-75%	50-75%	50-75%	50-75%
Study awareness and patient identification toolkits for sites	100%	100%	100%	100%	100%	100%	100%
Physician-to-patient letters/study awareness packets	50-75%	50-75%	50-75%	50-75%	50-75%	50-75%	50-75%
Physician education packages and follow-up mailers	50%	50%	50%	50%	50%	50%	50%
Physician outreach/education events	0-25%	0-25%	0-25%	0-25%	0-25%	0-25%	0-25%
Patient community/advocacy group outreach	50%	50%	50%	50%	50%	50%	50%
Study web site	N/A	50-75%	N/A	N/A	N/A	N/A	N/A
Web marketing	N/A	50-75%	N/A	N/A	N/A	N/A	N/A
Direct-to-patient advertising	N/A	0-25%	N/A	N/A	25-50%	N/A	N/A

Source: Ernst & Young, EMA, FDA and company web sites

be clearly explained so that everyone who is interested can understand the reasons for approving a particular medicine."

Arthur J. Higgins, CEO of Bayer Healthcare and EFPIA president, urged EC policymakers to use the economic crisis as an opportunity to re-think and modernize healthcare in Europe. EFPIA's vision, as characterized by Higgins, includes three main objectives:

1. to ensure swift and equal patient access to the best and safest medicines;
2. to achieve modern, efficient and sustainable healthcare systems; and
3. to support further development of innovation and medical programs.

In support of these objectives, Higgins said the European pharmaceutical industry is prepared to:

- Work harder to demonstrate the added value of innovations in a transparent manner that expedites access and removes roadblocks
- Develop high-quality, non-promotional information about disease treatments that enables patients to take a more active role in their health
- Increase the traceability of products, including a new coding system that reduces counterfeit medicines
- Get involved in more active dialogue in governments so, together, they can plan for innovation
- Partner with healthcare professionals to ensure medicines are used effectively, thereby reducing waste in the system.
- Further invest in R&D
- Commit to maintaining a strong industrial base in Europe, which will help the region bolster its image as a knowledge-based society
- Work with all stakeholders (i.e., EC, industry, companies, universities, regulatory agencies and patient organizations) to accelerate access to new medicines

In return, Higgins asked European governments to increase competition, create room for innovation, seek alternative sources of funding and recognize and reward innovation.

Author Biography

Over a career spanning more than 25 years, Dr. Diana Anderson-Foster, Ph.D., has helped pioneer best practices in patient recruitment and retention for global clinical trials—first as founder, president and CEO of D. Anderson & Company and today as president of DAC Patient Recruitment Services, an Imperial company. Her book credits include *International Patient Recruitment: Regulatory Guidelines, Customs and Practices*, *A Guide to Patient Recruitment* and *A Guide to Patient Recruitment and Retention*. In 2006, *PharmaVOICE* named her among the 100 Most Inspiring People in the Life Sciences Industry. She also received an International Women of Influence Award from the Global EXEC Women's International Council in 2008, among other honors.

References

1. *European Clinical Trial Site Options: An Insider's Analysis*, by Pavle Vukojevic, M.D. Published by Insight Pharma Reports, November 2008.
2. Hiddo J Lambers Heerspink, Daniela Dobre, Hans L Hillege, Diederick E Grobbee, and Dick de Zeeuw. *Does the European Clinical Trials Directive really improve clinical trial approval time?* Br J Clin Pharmacol.

2008 October; 66(4): 546–550.

3. Beyond Borders: Global Biotechnology Report 2011. 25th Anniversary edition. Ernst & Young.

4. European Federation of Pharmaceutical Industry Associations. Located online at www.efpia.eu/Content/Default.asp?PageID=358. Accessed September 2011.

5. European Federation of Pharmaceutical Industry Associations. Located online at www.efpia.eu/Content/Default.asp?PageID=573. Accessed September 2011.

CHAPTER SIXTEEN

Close Up on Central Europe

By Diana L. Anderson-Foster, Ph.D.

Central Europe (CE), also referred to as Middle Europe, is an expanse located between the diversely defined territories of Eastern and Western Europe. It stretches from the Baltic and North Sea to the north to the Adriatic Sea to the south and, according to the majority of sources, includes Austria, Czech Republic, Germany, Hungary, Liechtenstein, Poland, Slovakia, Slovenia and Switzerland. Other sources include Bulgaria and Romania as well. With a plethora of treatment-naive patients, lower saturation of competing trials and access to highly skilled investigators educated in the West, Central Europe holds great promise for life sciences companies conducting clinical trials.

Yet, despite its attractiveness, the region poses many challenges to pharmaceutical research and development. Clinical studies of all types are costly and time-consuming to conduct, often taking more than five years to complete. While Member States generally follow the European Clinical Trials Directive, varied interpretations yield country-specific differences that add to the complexity of trial execution across multiple jurisdictions. For example, in the U.K. conducting trials can be more bureaucratic and time-consuming, yielding high accountability but an overabundance of red tape. Other countries have similar systems but less red tape. Still, more countries, such as Germany, are becoming increasingly stringent in their processes.

Additionally, widespread recession has taken its toll on the region, as evidenced by record pharmacy closures and fewer drugs in the pipeline. Simultaneously, consumers are limiting their spending, businesses are keeping a tighter rein on costs and slowing Western markets are threatening exports. Contributing to this downturn are rising commodity prices, public debt levels, merger and acquisition activity, external global influences and foreign direct investment.

According to the European Federation of Pharmaceutical Industries and Associations (EFPIA), clinical innovation is essential to economic improvement in the region. However, in places such as Hungary, R&D expenditures are no longer tax-deductible, constituting a potential financial burden for large drug manufacturers.

Among struggling E.U. economies, Poland is a bright light, the only country to have avoided a recession. According to Eurasia analyst Eugene Chausovsky, Poland posted economic growth during 2008 and 2009, a time when countries such as France and Germany posted little to no growth. By the latest estimates, Poland is projected to grow at an annual rate of 4%.

Though progressive by comparison to its counterparts, Poland also has its pitfalls. In her report titled *Central European countries disinclined to boost consumption of innovative drugs*, pharmaceutical market analyst Agnieszka Stawarska noted there is no single legal act in force in Poland regulating the clinical research market.

"The relevant provisions pertaining to the clinical trials market are contained in various legal acts of various categories, including those relating solely to the pharmaceutical market (e.g. the Pharmaceutical Law), but also the Civil Code and the Penal Code," Stawarska wrote. "It is also worthy of note that provisions of various acts are frequently inconsistent with each other. In December 2009 the Ministry of Health published the assumptions underlying the Clinical Trials Act, but the act still has not come into force."

Regulatory aptitude is a prerequisite for successful clinical trial management from a patient recruitment and retention perspective. Over two decades, DAC Patient Recruitment Services has conducted training sessions and facilitated successful patient recruitment and retention programs in more than 100 countries, including those in Central Europe. DAC navigates world customs, regulations and cultural norms to provide country-level customization. Following is a case study of one such recruitment success story involving 37 non-U.S. sites, including Central Europe.

Case Study: Recruitment and Retention for Trial with Sites in Central Europe

Case Study stats

Indication: Rheumatoid arthritis (RA)

Number of sites: 42 (5 U.S.; 37 ROW)

Countries supported (13): Czech Republic, Hong Kong, Hungary, Russia, Serbia, Montenegro, Peru, Singapore, Slovakia, Spain, Taiwan, Turkey, Ukraine

Total number of patients: 85 (target=80)

Duration of service: 11 months

Global Management Strategies

DAC's overall recruitment campaign provided study sites with comprehensive, educational, patient-focused recruitment materials, internal study awareness materials and patient identification tools. These materials and tools were used to facilitate recruitment by helping study sites identify and screen patients faster, raise awareness among the staff and patients within their existing practices, and better educate referred patients to maximize the conversion rate to enrolled study participants. In addition, the recruitment program included a comprehensive recruitment-related training providing further recruitment information and support to both Pfizer and investigative sites.

DAC's direct-to-patient initiatives assisted with raising study awareness, enhancing understanding of clinical research and encouraging patients to explore study participation. These initiatives included community outreach among national and local patient advocacy and support groups, development of a study-specific web site and web marketing.

These direct activities, combined with other indirect study awareness activities, likely contributed to overall study awareness. DAC indirectly supported the enrollment of patients from within physicians' own practices and site databases by providing patient letters and recruitment materials for use by sites.

Program Objectives

The initial aim of the recruitment program was to support 41 U.S. and Rest-Of-World sites through an 11-month enrollment period. Upon awarding of the contract in June 2009, DAC provided services to augment the program, including patient-focused recruitment materials, internal study awareness

Figure 1: Project reporting structure

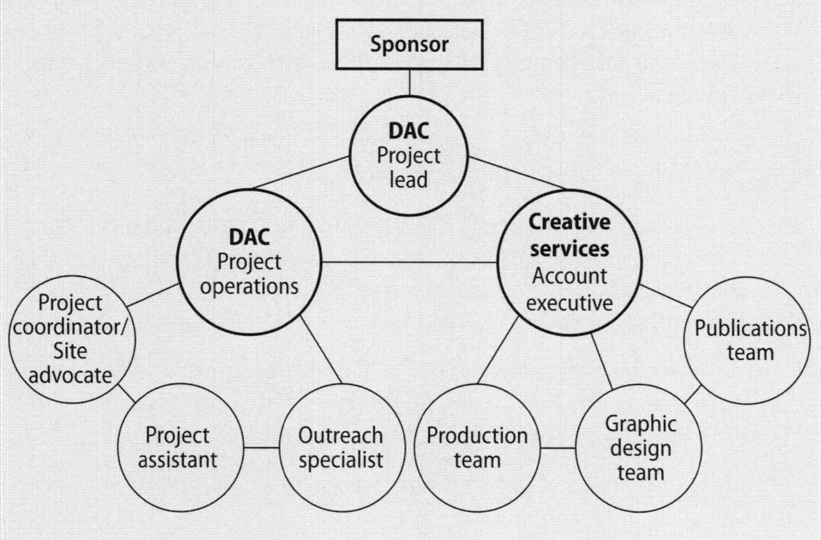

collateral and patient identification tools. The randomization target was 80 patients.

Program Strategies

DAC's overall recruitment campaign provided sites with tools to identify and screen patients faster, raise awareness among staff and patients and educate referred patients to facilitate their conversion to enrolled study participants. Specific elements included:

- Patient-focused recruitment materials
- Internal study awareness materials
- Patient identification tools
- Study web site and web marketing
- Patient community outreach
- Medical community outreach

Strategic Site Selection

The scope of DAC's involvement evolved to include site evaluation and identification of 20 investigators in: U.S., Czech Republic, Hong Kong, Hungary, Russia, Serbia, Slovakia, Spain, Taiwan and Turkey.

Service Descriptions

The comprehensive patient recruitment plan included the following initiatives. Among CE countries, site needs assessments revealed that patient referrals predominantly arise from internal sources. Materials provided to these sites were tailored accordingly, with an emphasis on physician education and study visit compliance.

Ready, Set, Recruit™ Recruitment Materials

Ready, Set, Recruit™ recruitment kits provided study sites with critical educational materials to increase study awareness and help RA patients and their families understand clinical research and study details.

Recruitment kits included:

- Study posters (two easel-backed for the waiting room and six wall posters) for use within the investigator's office, at recruitment events and/or in affiliated hospitals/facilities
- Study fliers (100) to foster patient awareness, generate interest and

prompt patients to seek more information

- Study brochures (100) with basic information as an introduction to the study; excellent tools for CRCs and investigators to use when first approaching a potential study participant
- Visit reminder appointment cards to keep the study fresh in the participant's mind, as well as aid compliance efforts
- Brochure holder (1)

All materials were customized with site-specific contact information and translated as necessary. Materials were sent to CRMs for distribution to sites.

Ready, Set, Recruit™ Patient Identification and Study Awareness Toolkits

Site toolkits containing internal awareness-building materials and patient identification aids further supported sites in their recruitment efforts. These tools helped study coordinators establish and maintain study awareness and aided in identifying potential participants.

Toolkits included:

- One staff-focused study poster for internal posting at the study site
- Five pocket protocols
- 10 inclusion/exclusion cards
- 100 chart review decals
- One pre-screening worksheet pad (100 worksheets per pad)
- One study procedure quick-reference flip book

These materials did not require IRB/EC approval.

Physician-to-Patient Study Awareness Packets and Follow-up Mailers

Targeted database searches and chart reviews to identify eligible patients in the sites' practices were essential to the recruitment effort. Educational physician-to-patient letters made outreach to pre-identified patients quick and easy for sites. Letter templates were provided on CD.

Packets included:

- One customized, site-specific physician-to-patient letter (available through the sponsor's study portal)
- One patient-focused study brochure
- One branded study magnet (with the study web site URL)

- One mailing envelope

The educational packets were sent at the launch of the recruitment program.

Physician-to-physician Education Packages

These materials provided potential referring physicians with essential study details for review to inform their decision to refer patients. Packages were designed for direct-mailings and/or distribution to each investigator's colleagues/contacts.

Packets included:

- One physician-to-physician referral letter (available through the sponsor's study portal)
- One physician-focused study brochure
- One I/E card
- One pre-screening/referral worksheets pad (25 sheets)
- One envelope

Follow-up study mailers served as a second mailing to potential referring physicians to reiterate study information and urge them to contact the site with any prospective referrals. Self-mailers were 8.5" x 14" quad-fold design printed in four-color. Follow-up mailers were sent two months after the initial educational packets were distributed.

Physician-Targeted Journal Advertising

To augment the study referral network, a physician-focused print advertisement was placed in rheumatology-related professional publications, such as

- *Arthritis & Rheumatism*
- *Clinical Rheumatology*
- *Rheumatology International.*

Each ad included the study email address. The assigned project lead coordinated physician inquires, and referrals were directed to the appropriate site.

Community Outreach and Grassroots Networking

Community outreach is an effective way for sites to create public awareness about clinical research in general and about their clinical research study in particular. It involves networking with professional organizations, patient advocates, patient support groups, community centers and physicians. Outreach activities can help clinical professionals raise awareness about their sites' ongoing studies while interfacing with prospective participants among clinical and patient populations.

As the sponsor's patient recruitment advocate with sites, DAC collaborated with country-specific CRAs to develop community outreach plans. DAC identified national organizations supporting RA patients within each country where the study was active. DAC contacted each organization/group to present study information, prepared and sent materials for distribution to the group's membership and placed study announcements in newsletters and on websites, as allowed.

In addition, in the U.S., DAC conducted outreach on both the national and local, site-specific level. At the site level, DAC identified and coordinated participation at local patient advocacy and support group events, including walks, fundraisers and support group meetings. DAC also secured distribution of materials and study information postings in newsletters and on web sites.

Study Web Site

An international study web site proved to be a key vehicle for accessing RA patients for the study.

The study web site included:

- A study overview
- Education on clinical research in general
- Answers to frequently asked questions
- A site locator. Site contact information was not listed on the web site; a "contact us form" allowed interested individuals to request more infor-

Figure 2: Enrollment progression projected vs. actual

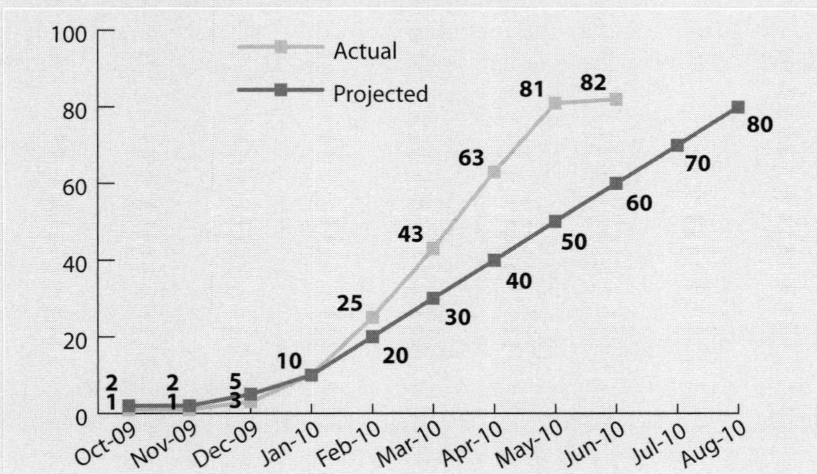

mation. The form was sent to DAC which, in turn, notified the site of required follow-up.

- A pre-screening option (U.S. only). The online pre-screening function permitted patients to identify themselves as potentially appropriate study participants.

The web site was presented in English, Spanish, Hungarian and Mandarin Chinese.

Program Evaluation

Enrollment targets were met three months ahead of schedule in May 2010, largely due to DAC's direct-to-patient initiatives, which raised study awareness, enhanced understanding of clinical research and encouraged patients to explore study participation.

As of May 31, 2010, 82 patients were randomized into the study due to joint efforts among the client, DAC and participating sites. A total of 208 patients were screened with 120 screen failures. The screen-failure rate for the duration of DAC's involvement averaged 57.7%.

Author Biography

Over a career spanning more than 25 years, Diana L. Anderson-Foster, Ph.D., has helped pioneer best practices in patient recruitment and retention for global clinical trials—first as founder, president and CEO of D. Anderson & Company and today as president of DAC Patient Recruitment Services, an Imperial company. Her book credits include *International Patient Recruitment: Regulatory Guidelines, Customs and Practices*, *A Guide to Patient Recruitment* and *A Guide to Patient Recruitment and Retention*. In 2006, *PharmaVOICE* named her among the 100 Most Inspiring People in the Life Sciences Industry. She also received an International Women of Influence Award from the Global EXEC Women's International Council in 2008, among other honors.

CHAPTER SEVENTEEN

Close Up on Latin America

By Dr. Marlene Llópiz

Introduction

The inhabitants of Latin America comprise a variety of ancestries, ethnic groups and races, making the region one of the most diverse in the world. Latin America consists of over 21 countries including Mexico and the Caribbean, as well as Central and South America. Clinical research is most prominent in Mexico, Argentina, Brazil, Chile and Colombia. Trials also are conducted in Venezuela, Peru and Uruguay in South America, and in Panama and Guatemala in Central America. Costa Rica also has been actively involved in clinical research for many years.

Clinical research in Latin America is not something new—nor is it any longer an "emerging region" when it comes to trial conduct. Clinical trials have been conducted ethically and professionally in Latin America for over 10 years.

However, certain characteristics of patients in each country must be carefully considered in order to understand how to optimize recruitment. These include:

- specific therapeutic indications and niches for emerging, neglected and seasonal diseases
- large ethnically diverse and naïve populations
- country age structure
- strong patient-doctor relationships
- good patient compliance and retention rates
- limited access to newly available and current state-of-the-art treatments
- motivated experienced investigators
- highly experienced monitoring and project management teams thoroughly trained on GCP and ICH guidelines
- a ready and professional supply of research sites and facilities.

Figure 1: Map of Latin America

Regions included in Latin America:

- Mexico
- Central America
- Caribbean
- South America

Clinical research takes place in:

- Mexico
- Argentina
- Guatemala
- Costa Rica
- Panama
- Colombia
- Venezuela
- Peru
- Chile
- Brazil

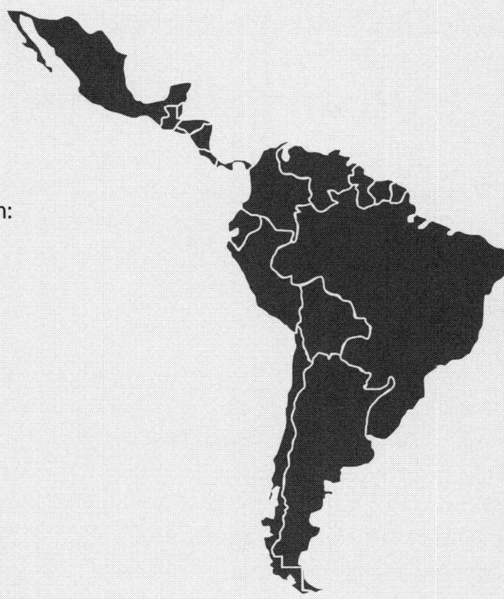

Although this chapter will focus on Mexico, Argentina and Brazil, other countries in the region will be referenced.

Regional Diseases and Therapeutic Indications

When a pharmaceutical or medical device company considers placing a trial in Latin America, the first step is finding a country that has a population with the specific disease to be studied. The disease may or may not be seasonal. Certain diseases occur at specific times of the year, depending on the location of the country—whether above or below the equator. Other diseases are totally unrelated to seasonal changes and occur throughout the year and in a substantial percent of the population. Nonetheless, a search for the right country with an adequate number of patients and the specified disease is essential for meeting recruitment expectations.

A first step recommended by most CROs is to conduct a feasibility study to locate an appropriate number of patients with the illness and seen by physicians at specific sites that have the necessary facilities for trial conduct. This often insures a step in the right direction for rapid patient recruitment. Nothing could be worse than starting a trial without insuring a minimal patient population with the necessary characteristics for complying with the study inclusion and exclusion criteria.

While Latin America is geographically situated in two hemispheres, it experiences seasonal diseases occurring at different times of the year. Planning enrollment based on seasonal differences helps maintain year-round patient enrollment and recruitment. Knowing the major causes of death and the incidence and prevalence of certain diseases gives each specific clinical trial an edge to better patient recruitment.

Latin America provides a large number of patients, both naïve to certain treatments as well as previously treated, who qualify for trial participation. Important sources for pinpointing specific diseases are incidence and prevalence rates often provided by governmental web sites. Sites specific for treating certain diseases serve as tertiary centers that may easily guarantee patients for trials.

Country Population Statistics

The total population for Latin America is close to 569 million—a more than sufficient number of patients for clinical trial conduct in many therapeutic indications. For example, Mexico has a population of 113,724,226 (July 2011 est. census). Brazil has 203,429,773 (July 2011 est.) inhabitants, while Argentina has 41,769,726 (July 2011 est.) people. Overall, 77% of the total Latin American population is concentrated in urban areas. The five largest cities are Mexico City, Mexico; Sao Paulo, Brazil; Buenos Aires, Argentina; Santiago, Chile; and Bogota, Colombia, with a combined population of over 58 million. These population densities can offer sponsors great advantages for patient recruitment and trial logistics, as fewer sites are necessary to achieve target patient populations. Equally important, a large percentage of this population qualifies as naïve subjects—who are increasingly difficult to find and recruit elsewhere.[1, 2, 3]

Mexico

In Mexico, the 10 major causes of death are coronary heart disease, diabetes mellitus, cerebrovascular disease (stroke), cirrhosis and chronic liver diseases, chronic obstructive pulmonary disease (COPD), motor vehicle or road traffic accidents, lower acute respiratory infections, violence (homicide), hypertensive heart disease and kidney failure.

This can be broken down further by gender and age, specifying exactly which groups are more vulnerable to certain diseases. For example, breast cancer is currently the leading cause of death among Mexican women, followed by cervical cancer. Each year, 13,000 Mexicans are diagnosed with breast cancer, the equivalent of 35 per day. Approximately 5,000 women are dying from this disease annually in the country. Breast cancer is a serious

Figure 2: Top 50 causes of death in Mexico

Per 100,000 population

		Deaths	%			Deaths	%
1	Coronary heart disease	77,045	16.09	26	Leukemia	4,096	0.86
2	Diabetes mellitus	71,906	15.02	27	Pancreas cancer	3,943	0.82
3	Stroke	34,267	7.16	28	Lymphomas	3,937	0.82
4	Liver disease	28,324	5.92	29	Diarrheal diseases	3,728	0.78
5	Lung disease	22,884	4.78	30	Birth trauma	3,111	0.65
6	Violence	19,476	4.07	31	Peptic ulcer disease	2,929	0.61
7	Hypertension	17,838	3.73	32	Tuberculosis	2,665	0.56
8	Influenza and pneumonia	16,535	3.45	33	Alzheimer´s/ dementia	2,615	0.55
9	Road traffic accidents	13,754	2.87	34	Anemia	2,536	0.53
10	Kidney disease	13,591	2.84	35	Drowning	2,521	0.53
11	Other injuries	13,456	2.81	36	Falls	2,405	0.50
12	Congenital anomalies	9,386	1.96	37	Asthma	1,792	0.37
13	Endocrine disorders	9,370	1.96	38	Ovary cancer	1,761	0.37
14	Malnutrition	8,947	1.87	39	Maternal conditions	1,743	0.36
15	Lung cancer	7,343	1.53	40	Epilepsy	1,671	0.35
16	Low birth weight	6,697	1.40	41	Skin disease	1,580	0.33
17	Stomach cancer	6,390	1.33	42	Inflammatory/heart	1,555	0.32
18	Prostate cancer	6,101	1.27	43	Skin cancer	1,523	0.32
19	Liver cancer	5,501	1.15	44	Rheumatoid arthritis	1,411	0.29
20	Breast cancer	5,383	1.12	45	Bladder cancer	1,237	0.26
21	HIV/AIDS	5,143	1.07	46	Poisonings	1,234	0.26
22	Suicide	4,764	1.00	47	Parkinson disease	1,224	0.26
23	Colorectal cancer	4,672	0.98	48	Rheumatic heart disease	1,133	0.24
24	Cervical cancer	4,464	0.93	49	Oral cancer	1,078	0.23
25	Other neoplasms	4,283	0.89	50	Esophageal cancer	1,075	0.22

Source: www.worldlifeexpectancy.com/country-health-profile/mexico

threat to the health of women globally and an unrecognized priority in middle-income countries.[4]

Breast cancer accounts for more deaths than cervical cancer since 2006; it is the second cause of death for women ages 30 to 54. Data on detection, although under-reported, show 6,000 new cases in 1990 and a projected increase to over 16,500 per year by 2020. This is very important when considering the incidence rate for new cases and treatment options for women. Further, the majority of breast cancer cases are self-detected, and only 10% of all cases are detected in stage one. Better and earlier detection methods, as well as newer and better treatments for later stages, are required. Mexico's social security systems cover approximately 40% to 45% of the population and include breast cancer treatment. As of 2007, the rest of the population has the right to breast cancer treatment through Popular Health Insurance ("Seguro Popular"). Despite these entitlements, services are lacking and interventions for early detection, particularly mammography, are very limited.

New treatments for breast cancer and clinical trials are an important niche for pharmaceutical companies to market innovative drugs. There are a sufficient amount of patients for expedite patient recruitment and treatment.[5]

Overall, trials related to any of these diseases offering therapeutic solutions would be successful in Mexico. The epidemiology behind each disease in the different countries provides a clear picture as to the success of a trial when patients with the specific diseases are available for patient recruitment.

Figure 3: Cancer ranking by type for Mexico

Per 100,000 population

		Rate	World rank			Rate	World rank
1	Breast cancer	11.34	156	**10**	Lymphomas	4.42	121
2	Lung cancer	8.59	116	**11**	Leukemia	4.13	78
3	Stomach cancer	7.31	85	**12**	Ovarian cancer	1.99	108
4	Prostate cancer	7.07	80	**13**	Skin cancer	1.72	66
5	Liver cancer	6.41	86	**14**	Bladder cancer	1.43	135
6	Colorectal cancer	5.35	127	**15**	Esophageal cancer	1.26	153
7	Cervical cancer	4.98	101	**16**	Oral cancer	1.24	180
8	Other neoplasms	4.76	39	**17**	Uterine cancer	0.81	112
9	Pancreas cancer	4.61	66				

Source: www.worldlifeexpectancy.com/country-health-profile/mexico

Figure 4: 2010 Population by age and gender, Mexico

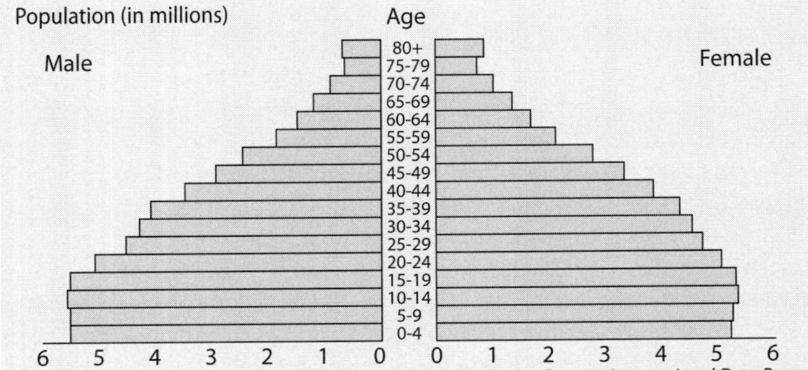

Source: U.S. Census Bureau, International Data Base

Age Structure

The age structure for Mexico's population is as follows:

- **0-14 years:** 28.2% (male 16,395,974/female 15,714,182)
- **15-64 years:** 65.2% (male 35,842,495/female 38,309,528)
- **65 and over:** 6.6% (male 3,348,495/female 4,113,552) (2011 est.) [1,6]

The importance of these figures lies in knowing your target population for a specific disease based on gender and age distribution.

Argentina

In Argentina, coronary heart disease is the leading cause of death, followed by stroke, influenza and pneumonia, lung cancer, diabetes mellitus, colon and rectal cancer and kidney disease. Heart disease, cerebrovascular diseases and malignant tumors were the leading causes of death among both sexes in the last few years.

According to official figures, for some decades complications from illegal abortion are considered the leading cause of maternal death in Argentina.[7]

When specifically looking at the different types of cancers affecting Argentina, breast cancer takes the lead, followed by lung, colorectal, prostate, pancreatic, stomach and lymphomas.

Age Structure

The age structure for Argentina is as follows:

- **0-14 years:** 25.4% (male 5,429,488/female 5,181,289)
- **15-64 years:** 63.6% (male 13,253,468/female 13,301,530)
- **65 and over:** 11% (male 1,897,144/female 2,706,807) (2011 est.) [3,8]

Figure 5: Top 50 causes of death in Argentina

Per 100,000 population

		Deaths	%			Deaths	%
1	Coronary heart disease	36,415	16.76	**26**	Esophageal cancer	2,322	1.07
2	Stroke	22,859	10.52	**27**	Cervical cancer	2,215	1.02
3	Influenza and pneumonia	20,366	9.37	**28**	Leukemia	2,044	0.94
4	Lung cancer	10,033	4.62	**29**	Liver cancer	2,000	0.92
5	Diabetes mellitus	8,911	4.10	**30**	Bladder cancer	1,651	0.76
6	Colon-rectal cancer	8,575	3.95	**31**	HIV/AIDS	1,572	0.72
7	Kidney disease	7,807	3.59	**32**	Skin disease	1,485	0.68
8	Other injuries	7,403	3.41	**33**	Malnutrition	1,282	0.59
9	Breast cancer	6,702	3.08	**34**	Ovary cancer	1,232	0.57
10	Hypertension	6,487	2.99	**35**	Oral cancer	1,072	0.49
11	Lung disease	5,078	2.34	**36**	Skin cancers	973	0.45
12	Prostate cancer	4,974	2.29	**37**	Uterine cancer	884	0.41
13	Road traffic accidents	4,880	2.25	**38**	Parkinson´s disease	877	0.40
14	Pancreas cancer	4,343	2.00	**39**	Birth trauma	840	0.39
15	Suicide	3,707	1.71	**40**	Alcohol	732	0.34
16	Stomach cancer	3,651	1.68	**41**	Tuberculosis	681	0.31
17	Alzheimer´s/dementia	3,599	1.66	**42**	Drowning	650	0.30
18	Inflammatory/heart	3,506	1.61	**43**	Asthma	589	0.27
19	Endocrine disorders	3,102	1.43	**44**	Maternal conditions	519	0.24
20	Congenital anomalies	3,025	1.39	**45**	Fires	507	0.23
21	Liver disease	3,000	1.38	**46**	Chagas disease	448	0.21
22	Other neoplasms	2,864	1.32	**47**	Meningitis	415	0.19
23	Lymphomas	2,665	1.23	**48**	Diarrheal diseases	408	0.19
24	Low birth weight	2,660	1.22	**49**	Anemia	406	0.19
25	Violence	2,465	1.13	**50**	Peptic ulcer disease	387	0.18

Source: www.worldlifeexpectancy.com/country-health-profile/argentina

Figure 6: Cancer ranking by type for Argentina

Per 100,000 population

		Rate	World rank			Rate	World rank
1	Breast cancer	24.83	15	10	Esophageal cancer	4.75	52
2	Lung cancer	21.76	51	11	Leukemia	4.41	60
3	Colorectal cancer	17.12	22	12	Liver cancer	4.09	136
4	Prostate cancer	9.13	47	13	Bladder cancer	3.17	63
5	Pancreas cancer	8.76	13	14	Ovarian cancer	2.65	66
6	Stomach cancer	7.60	81	15	Oral cancer	2.34	116
7	Other neoplasms	5.99	15	16	Skin cancers	2.01	49
8	Lymphomas	5.71	78	17	Uterine cancer	1.75	49
9	Cervical cancer	5.17	97				

Source: www.worldlifeexpectancy.com/country-health-profile/argentina

Figure 7: 2010 Population by age and gender, Argentina

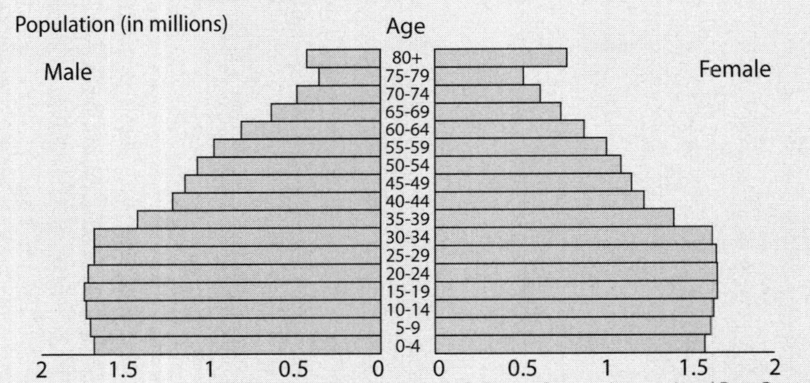

Source: U.S. Census Bureau, International Data Base

Brazil

Coronary heart disease is the top cause of death in Brazil, followed by stroke, diabetes mellitus, influenza and pneumonia, violence, hypertension, lung disease, road vehicle accidents, lung cancer and liver disease.

The main cancer types are lung and breast, followed by stomach, prostate, colorectal, cervical, liver and esophageal cancer.

Age Structure

For Brazil, the age structure is as follows:

- **0-14 years:** 26.2% (male 27,219,651/female 26,180,040)
- **15-64 years:** 67% (male 67,524,642/female 68,809,357)
- **65 and over:** 6.7% (male 5,796,433/female 7,899,650) (2011 est.) [2,9]

Doctor-Patient Relationship

Each Latin American country has a unique culture despite its close geographic proximity to its neighboring countries. Knowing those differences will allow sponsors greater success in trial conduct and patient recruitment. A lesson learned is that even though the countries are all in Latin America, each country's population is uniquely different. Two languages are spoken—Spanish, in most countries, and Portuguese, spoken in Brazil.

Study participants are very keen in identifying competent, personable and experienced recruiters to positively influence their decision to participate in research. As in other regions, Latin Americans hold great trust in their physicians and nurses. How they are treated will influence their desire to take part in and remain in trials. Patient retention is often a problem of distance and cost—not adverse events or lack of desire to participate. Properly explaining studies, describing procedures in detail and speaking to patients in a clear language they understand while answering their questions is of extreme importance to patients. Clarity and orderly study conduct help patients to adhere to and comply with the rules for trial follow through.

For example, while most principal investigators can speak English, the ability of a sponsor´s representative to communicate in Spanish (or Portuguese) is helpful to establish positive communication and respect within native populations. Although most trials are conducted through CROs, clear communication is of the essence between sponsors, principal investigators, CRO and study staff. The staff has to have a clear line of communication with patients to insure patient recruitment and retention.

The first step investigators must take as they prepare to recruit study participants is to develop a relevant definition of the subject populations as per the study protocol. The protocol details the necessary patient characteristics. Adequate and timely participant recruitment can determine a research

Figure 8: Top 50 causes of death in Brazil

Per 100,000 population

		Deaths	%			Deaths	%
1	Coronary heart disease	133,992	13.76	26	Liver cancer	8,907	0.91
2	Stroke	123,034	12.63	27	Alcohol	8,523	0.88
3	Diabetes mellitus	61,987	6.36	28	Malnutrition	8,468	0.87
4	Influenza and pneumonia	60,951	6.26	29	Esophageal cancer	7,999	0.82
5	Violence	56,841	5.84	30	Oral cancer	7,650	0.79
6	Hypertension	53,466	5.49	31	Birth trauma	7,404	0.76
7	Lung disease	43,373	4.45	32	Pancreas cancer	7,071	0.73
8	Road traffic accidents	42,071	4.32	33	Lymphomas	7,029	0.72
9	Lung cancer	22,747	2.34	34	Drowning	6,796	0.70
10	Liver disease	22,731	2.33	35	Diarrheal diseases	6,785	0.70
11	Inflammatory/heart	19,315	1.98	36	Leukemia	6,679	0.69
12	Stomach cancer	16,832	1.73	37	Chagas disease	6,247	0.64
13	Kidney disease	15,350	1.58	38	Tuberculosis	5,577	0.57
14	Other injuries	15,023	1.54	39	Peptic ulcer disease	3,961	0.41
15	Prostate cancer	14,428	1.48	40	Other neoplasms	3,753	0.39
16	HIV/AIDS	14,361	1.47	41	Asthma	3,396	0.35
17	Endocrine disorders	14,081	1.45	42	Skin disease	3,366	0.35
18	Alzheimer´s/dementia	13,818	1.42	43	Bladder cancer	3,201	0.33
19	Congenital anomalies	12,851	1.32	44	Ovary cancer	2,982	0.31
20	Breast cancer	12,573	1.29	45	Rheumatic heart disease	2,974	0.31
21	Colorectal cancer	11,763	1.21	46	Parkinson disease	2,835	0.29
22	Falls	11,490	1.18	47	Anemia	2,568	0.26
23	Low birth weight	11,396	1.17	48	Epilepsy	2,515	0.26
24	Cervical cancer	11,055	1.13	49	Hepatitis C	2,453	0.25
25	Suicide	10,980	1.13	50	Skin cancers	2,219	0.23

Source: www.worldlifeexpectancy.com/country-health-profile/brazil

Figure 9: Cancer ranking by type for Brazil

Per 100,000 population

		Rate	World rank			Rate	World rank
1	Lung cancer	13.96	89	10	Pancreas cancer	4.32	72
2	Breast cancer	13.65	124	11	Lymphomas	4.17	126
3	Stomach cancer	10.21	53	12	Leukemia	3.80	102
4	Prostate cancer	9.00	49	13	Other neoplasms	2.22	122
5	Colon-rectal cancer	7.09	95	14	Bladder cancer	1.96	104
6	Cervical cancer	6.45	81	15	Ovary cancer	1.78	130
7	Liver cancer	5.41	102	16	Skin cancers	1.31	89
8	Esophageal cancer	4.84	51	17	Uterine cancer	1.25	82
9	Oral cancer	4.56	49				

Source: www.worldlifeexpectancy.com/country-health-profile/brazil

Figure 10: 2010 Population by age and gender, Brazil

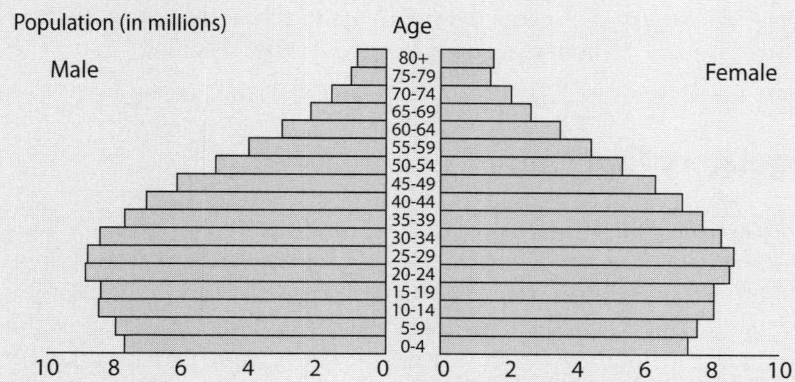

Source: U.S. Census Bureau, International Data Base

study's success. Enrolling a targeted sample size during a specified time period helps ensure sufficient statistical power and keeps study operations within budget, time and personnel constraints.

Most patients in Latin America happily take part in clinical trials. Often, the medical services available to patients are insufficient and deficient. Participating in trials offers additional benefits and insures patients' continuous testing, checkups, medication and more personalized treatment.

In some Latin American countries, such as Mexico, patients cannot be offered payment for taking part in trials. However, providing meals or monetary help for transportation can be offered to ease the burden of complying with appointments or traveling from distant towns to medical centers or sites.

Access to New and State-of-the-Art Treatments

In Latin America, the majority of patient populations receive healthcare and treatment from governmental institutions, and others use physicians at private practices and hospitals. Whether trials are conducted at either type of institution, patients receive more personalized care while participating in clinical trials.

Latin America has a large number of drug naïve patients. Often, patients have not had the opportunity to be treated with state-of-the-art drugs for specific diseases, such as different types of cancers. These drugs have not reached Latin America—thus the need for clinical trials to bring these treatments to market in these countries. Latin America offers sponsors an advantage to test drugs in patients who are naïve to treatments, to ensure the treatments work without a previous history of other schemes.

Regulatory Timelines

Timelines are of vital importance for the development of a new drug. Too often, Latin American nations are considered for involvement at the last minute when planning a trial. It is important to stress that Latin American countries should not be considered "rescue countries" for clinical trial conduct. The time spent waiting for patient recruitment in other nations and often not met within the stipulated timelines could be used for regulatory approval processes in Latin America. These processes typically average from 10 to 14 weeks—longer than in North America but not longer than some European countries. The average timeline for approvals in Latin America is three to four months from the time the final protocol is translated into Spanish and/or Portuguese to the start of the study.

Clinical trial conduct in Latin America is considered at times a good "second choice" when recruitment is deficient and scarce in other regions of the world. The belief that regulatory timelines are lengthy is often reconsidered when expedited recruitment is needed.

Early planning should include a strategy for site selection that balances each country's regulatory approval time, patient recruitment potential and site capabilities. It often is worthwhile to spend time analyzing the possibility of investing in a trial in Latin America from the start and take the first steps in regulatory submissions, than add these countries once a global trial has begun. The planning process must include a review of the most current regulatory procedures, drug importation and other issues to ensure that expectations are appropriately set before trials begin. In addition, focusing on the five major Latin American cities and the tertiary sites where patients are pooled is crucial.

Often, these timeline differences are not considered during development planning. Latin America as part of a global study may not be considered feasible. This can leave sponsors with an incorrect impression regarding Latin American trial capabilities because they do not have an opportunity to take advantage of the rapid patient recruitment and higher patient retention that offset longer regulatory approval. According to a recent survey, only 41% of clinical trials conducted at Latin American sites have more than a one month delay in enrollment, compared with 55% at European sites and 70% at U.S. sites.

Most countries have strict regulations for the import of drug supplies and the export of biological materials such as subject samples. A partner with expertise in local customs regulations to aid in the review of import documents ahead of study supply shipments, as well as the capability to facilitate the local distribution, can save considerable time and help avoid customs delays. Mexico, for example, has included the importation/exportation permit within its approval process when authorization is granted by the Ministry of Health.[10, 11]

Informed Consent and Ethics Approval

One very important cultural difference between studies in the U.S. and Latin America is the informed consent form (ICF). The most common reason for regulatory delays in clinical trials is due to problems with the ICF, which can be avoided with proper preparation. Many sponsors overestimate the education level of the population, and regulatory authorities will often reject translations of approved ICF forms originating from countries with more educated populations, such as the U.S. The level of information most sponsors require from their ICF needs to be readdressed, especially for trials that involve complex procedures that can confuse a patient's decision.

In Mexico, for example, while most health institutions follow informed consent procedures recommended by international pharmaceutical companies and that have FDA approval, they usually request subjects sign a simpler consent form written in a basic language and requiring the signatures of two additional witnesses. In pediatric trials, the parents or guardians must sign the form and, when age permits, adolescents sign an acceptance form.

One way to avoid these delays and speed patient recruitment is to revise the original ICF in English in a simpler language for patients to understand, including the two witnesses and any additional information that must be included, before the ICF is translated into Spanish. This way the sponsor views exactly what will be translated and the ethics committees and health authorities will be satisfied with its content.

In addition to the standard risk/benefit assessment, Latin American ethics committees focus on beneficence for patients and carefully evaluate the healthcare context and social situation of the potential subjects. The use of placebo, payment for participation, consent process and the expectation of post-study treatment may be required to achieve ethics approval.

Experienced Monitoring, Project Management Teams

CROs have flourished in Latin America and become key strategic partners to most pharmaceutical and biotech companies. This kind of alliance allows sponsors to concentrate on their core skills, mostly in manufacturing, marketing and sales. It is more convenient and time-saving for pharmaceutical and device companies to outsource tasks such as regulatory submissions, patient recruitment, project management and clinical monitoring. Most of the time, CROs offer recommended sites for sponsors. These sites should be high recruiters—within time and budget—and certainly of the highest quality.

The growing success of the pharmaceutical business in the region reflects the significant investments made in Latin America by most of the world's major pharmaceutical companies, as well as the presence of numerous CROs and other companies, such as organized recruitment firms, that supply support services to the pharmaceutical industry. The availability of these resources in turn supports the growth of clinical trials in the region.

Conclusion

The rapid growth of the pharmaceutical market in Latin America is likely to continue due to estimates in population growth. This in turn supports the growth of clinical trials in the region, which has tremendous untapped potential and capacity for trials. Latin America's advantages as a location for clinical trials are confirmed by the hundreds of ICH-compliant trials already successfully conducted or underway.

Latin American clinical trial growth occurs not only because of its reputation for high recruitment of treatment-naïve patients, but also due to increased recognition of the region´s contribution to scientific research with high-quality standards and patient recruitment.

Author Biography

Marlene Llópiz is president of the AMEIFAC-Mexico, the Association of Medical Specialists in the Pharmaceutical Industry for the 2011-2013 tenure. She is Secretary General for IFAPP, the International Federation of Association of Pharmaceutical Physicians. Marlene holds a B.A. in biochemistry from Austin College, an M.D. from Universidad Anahuac and her MPH from the Harvard School of Public Health (Clinical Effectiveness). She is chief executive officer of Clinica Responsable Operativa, a consulting agency in clinical affairs for Latin America.

References

1. www.indexmundi.com/mexico/demographics_profile.html
2. www.indexmundi.com/brazil/demographics_profile.html
3. www.indexmundi.com/argentina/demographics_profile.html
4. www.hispanicallyspeakingnews.com/notitas-de-noticias/details/mexico-tackling-breast-cancer-a-leading-cause-of-death-for-women/11048/
5. Knaul FM, Nigenda G, Lozano R et al. *Breast cancer in Mexico: a pressing priority. Reproductive Health Matters* Vol. 16, Issue 32, pp. 113-123.
6. www.nationmaster.com/country/mx-mexico/Age-_distribution
7. http://abortionnews.info/article/Argentina-to-Tackle-500000-Annual-Abortions-that-Take-Place--Leading-Cause-of----
8. www.nationmaster.com/country/ar-argentina/Age-_distribution
9. www.nationmaster.com/country/br-brazil/Age-_distribution
10. www.wipro.com/Documents/TW_1108035_StofClinTrials_REV_v1.pdf
11. www.theoremclinical.com/Userfiles/Docs/ICTLATAMSpring2011 Omnicare.pdf

CHAPTER EIGHTEEN

Close Up on India

By Dan McDonald

In recent years, there has been tremendous publicity regarding the significant movement of clinical trials to emerging markets such as Brazil, Russia, India and China, the "BRIC" countries. Large, often treatment-naïve patient populations, western-trained physician investigators and improving regulatory environments all made these countries much more attractive for sponsors looking to accelerate enrollment and reduce costs.

Unfortunately, despite the claims, successfully recruiting, enrolling and retaining patients present unique challenges in these countries. It is not simply a matter of receiving regulatory approval and contracting sites. Instead, successful recruitment and retention, particularly in India, requires critical knowledge development, including ethics committee approvals for certain recruitment strategies, identification and selection of qualified sites, understanding of cultural and socioeconomic factors and, perhaps most importantly, strong local expertise. Local expertise can be achieved only through strong experience and ground-based infrastructure, personnel and resources.

The business of global patient recruitment has become highly professionalized and sophisticated. Patient Recruitment Organizations (PROs) have developed new technologies and processes that allow sponsors to intelligently and accurately identify patients, forecast enrollment rates and execute strategies better than ever. Despite these advances, clinical trial protocols are becoming more complex, sample size requirements are growing and sponsors and PROs are being forced outside their mature market comfort zone to emerging markets, where different rules apply. Unlike mature markets, emerging markets such as India require much more traditional, ground-based, grassroots strategies, based less on technology and more on proper planning, resource allocation and hard work.

In fact, an ongoing survey conducted by Excel Life Sciences of more than 1,000 study volunteers in India demonstrates this point. The survey found 97% of trial volunteers first learned about a clinical trial through a physician: 67% through their own physician and 30% through another physician. This differs dramatically from the U.S., where nearly 70% of patients go outside their managed care organization and self-refer into a trial after learning

Figure 1: Importance of site management

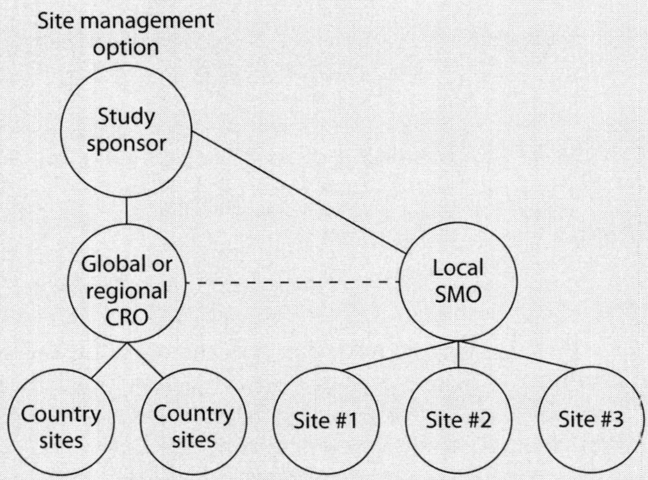

- Large sites, significant patient loads leave PIs with little time
- Site-employed CRCs don't exist or are spread thin
- Provides critical day-to-day support to ensure study runs smoothly, correctly, ethically and transparently
- Well-tested operating processes
- Creation and implementation of site working practice documents/SOPs
- Use of communication technology to ensure compliance
- Ensures IRB submissions completed properly and queries addressed
- Provides safeguard to ensure GCP compliance
- Positively affects enrollment rates, retention rates and data quality
- Ensures patients have support system

Source: Excel Life Sciences 2010 analysis of service provider operating models used by trial sponsors in India

about it through the Internet, advertising or media campaigns.

This chapter includes several case studies and tips on successful patient recruitment and retention in India that can be applied to other emerging markets, and highlights the creative thinking, strategic planning and unique operating models that can be used to meet study objectives.

Unique Market Characteristics for Consideration

Many elements of the Indian market for clinical research must be taken into account when planning a recruitment and retention strategy. While an entire book could be dedicated just to this topic, some of the more important elements are captured below and should be considered before starting a study in India:

- **97% of study subjects first learn of a clinical trial through their primary care physician or another physician.**
  - Selection of the right sites is critical to the success of the study.
  - Development and execution of a robust physician referral program should be a recruitment strategy for nearly all applicable studies.
- **On average, physicians see more than 50 and as many as 100 patients per day at their practices.**
  - Consider posting notices about the study in public areas.
  - Provide investigators and other potential referring physicians with pocket cheat cards printed with the study criteria.
- **Less than 15% of investigative sites have a full-time study coordinator. When a coordinator is present, that individual is often responsible for managing multiple studies.**
  - Given patient loads and the low occurrence of proper on-site coordinator support, consider the use of a site management organization in India.
  - The operating model of some SMOs in India includes the placement of a highly trained clinical research coordinator at each study site. The economies of scale in India allow for that coordinator to be dedicated to a single sponsor study and provide critical day-to-day support to the investigators, who are busy seeing patients.
  - Study coordinators provided by an SMO will assist the investigator with several critical activities related to recruitment and retention, including:

    Pre-study:

    - Patient database review and pre-screening
    - Identify physician network
    - Initiate contact with referring physicians and evaluate patient database

    Study conduct:

    - Assist in ICF process
    - Track enrollment
    - Ensure 100% follow up
    - Issue timely payments for patient expenses

- Ensure subject compliance with electronic diary requirements
- Execute patient recruitment strategies
- Plan and conduct physician lunches
- Develop community outreach programs
- Provide patient visit reminders and transportation assistance

- **Potential study patients rarely attend a screening visit alone. In fact, in the survey of study volunteers in India by Excel Life Sciences, only 8% made the decision to participate on their own, versus 38% in the U.S. Most patients attend the screening visits with a loved one or caretaker.**
  - Be prepared to address both the patient and his or her attendant during the study introduction conversation and study consenting process. A patient and caregiver information sheet or brochure can be useful to ensure everyone's questions are answered and patients understand the risks and requirements associated with participation.
  - This unique element of the Indian culture can make the initial consenting process a little tedious, but there are benefits. With patients' loved ones and caregivers participating in the scrutinous decision process, patients seem to make more informed choices to participate. This, combined with the additional support provided by the on-site dedicated clinical reseach coordinator, has resulted in retention rates above 90% versus the industry average of only 75%.
  - These factors also resulted in a strong understanding of the study requirements and expectations, according to the study volunteer survey:

Figure 2: Who assisted with patient's decision?

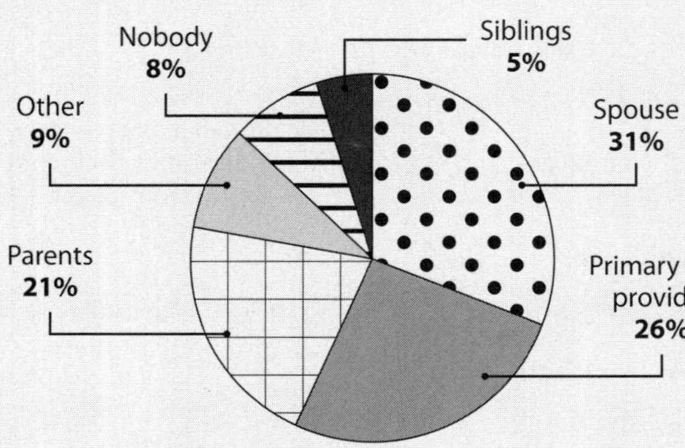

Source: Excel Life Sciences 2010 Informed Consent and Volunteer Experience Survey–India

- 98% understood the number of times they would have to visit the site
- 93% understood that the study would carry risks and discomforts
- 56% were unaware of clinical research prior to participating in a study
- 97% understood the informed consent form (70% very well; 27% well)

- **Hindi is the official language of the Republic of India, while English is the second official language.** Nearly all physicians, nurses and hospital administrators speak fluent English. In addition to these languages, at least 29 languages are spoken by more than one million people, while 122 are spoken by more than 10,000. Fortunately, the language of global clinical research trials in India is English, and all regulatory documents are submitted in English.
  - ICF and patient information sheets need to be translated into five languages on average for each study. Any other patient-facing materials also must be translated.

Figure 3: Patient understanding, U.S. vs. India

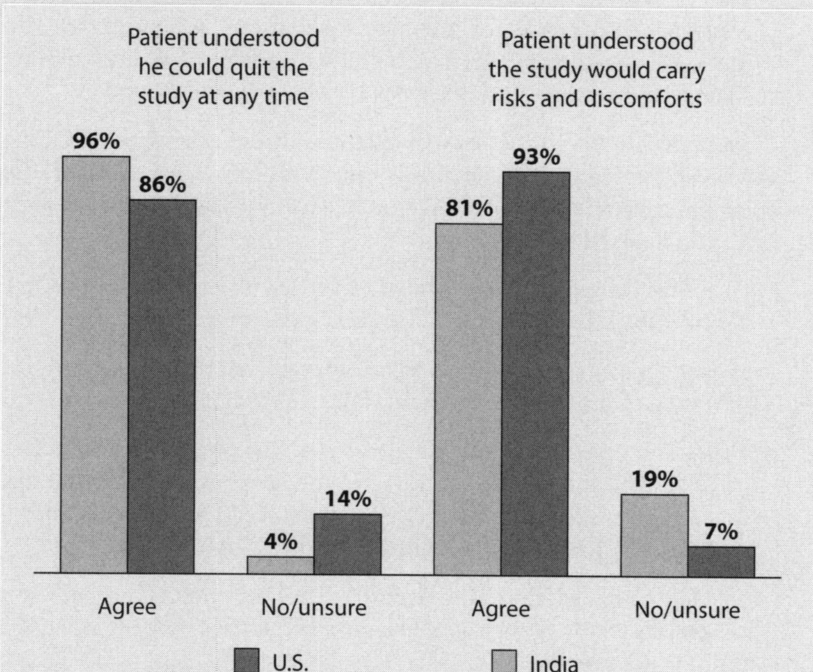

Source: Excel Life Sciences 2010 Informed Consent and Volunteer Experience Survey–India; CenterWatch 2006 National Survey of Study Volunteer Experiences–U.S.

  - If using an SMO and dedicated clinical research coordinator, make sure the coordinator is from the local area and can speak the most common languages or dialects to ensure proper communication with study subjects.

- **Clinical research is largely unknown across India and only an estimated 30,000 of India's 1.2 billion patients have participated in clinical trials.**
  - Recruitment materials need to include not only information about the study but also basic information about the clinical trials process.

- **Many study subjects will need to travel one to three hours to reach the study site. Most of these patients will be accompanied by an attendant. Most will travel via public transportation.**
  - Select sites that are convenient to public transportation.
  - A small stipend should be included in the study budget for both the patient and attendant.

- **India has nearly 900 million mobile phone subscribers as of the summer of 2011. Most people have a mobile phone and not a land line, and texting is a popular and acceptable method of communicating.**
  - For retention of patients and compliance with study requirements, consider text messages for following up about upcoming study visits, including alerting patients to take study medications and reminding them to complete their diaries.

- **Most recruitment strategies will require Ethics Committee (EC) approval. Typically, ECs meet only once a month. While central ECs exist, most sites have a local EC that has jurisdiction over what strategies can be used at that site.**
  - Given the infrequency with which ECs meet, it's important to collect the meeting schedule of the EC at each site as early as possible.
  - Proper planning is required to ensure that all materials and descriptions of strategies and use are ready in advance of the next EC meeting.
  - Don't wait until the EC meeting to alert an investigator (and EC if possible) about the types of strategies you are considering. Make sure to ask the investigator what strategies they would recommend and which strategies have been approved by the EC in the past.
  - The following diagram lists other strategies you might consider using, the commonality of their use, likelihood of approval by the EC and typical effectiveness.

Figure 4: Consideration of common enrollment strategies in India

Dear colleague letters

- High usage
- EC approval required
- 100% probability of EC approval
- Very effective

Physician awareness packets

- Medium usage
- EC approval required
- 75% probability of EC approval
- Effective

Physician luncheons

- Medium usage
- EC approval required
- 50% probability of EC approval
- Effective

Patient awareness and educational materials

- Low usage
- EC approval required
- 50% probability of EC approval
- Somewhat effective

Community outreach

- Medium usage
- No EC approval required
- Very effective

Public advertising

- Low/rare usage
- EC approval required
- <25% probability of EC approval
- Effectiveness unkown

Caregiver awareness and educational materials

- Low usage
- EC approval required
- 25% probability of EC approval
- Somewhat effective

Source: The Importance of a Strong Study Feasibility Process, Accurate Site Selection and Patient Enrollment Strategy in India. S Das, Director of Operations and Country Head, Excel Life Sciences at the "ACRP 2009 Global Conference and Exhibition" Denver, CO, April 2009

Other Items for Consideration in Study Planning

- Most people are treatment naïve compared to Western standards, and alternative medicine is common.
- Only 25% of India's population has access to Western medicine (allopathic), practiced mainly in urban areas.
- Roughly 11% of India's population has health insurance, with only 2% to 3% having private health insurance.

Case Studies

Consideration of unique demographic, socio-economic and cultural intricacies in study feasibility and patient enrollment

Scenario:

Sponsor:	Asia Pacific-based multinational
Phase:	III
Condition:	Ovarian Carcinoma of Epithelial Origin
Target patients:	Late-stage, histologically-confirmed, platinum-resistant
Countries:	7 (Including India)
Sites:	7 in India (60–80 globally)

An Asia Pacific-based global pharmaceutical company was in the early stages of conducting a multinational clinical trial targeting ovarian cancer. The company was experiencing significant recruitment challenges in other parts of the world and was, therefore, considering India as a destination for some study sites. As is becoming increasingly common, the study sponsor was requiring the country-specific trial management organization to conduct a feasibility analysis using only a draft protocol, of which several key eligibility criteria were missing. This presented a unique opportunity for an analysis of the impact some of the demographic, socio-economic and cultural intricacies of an emerging market such as India can have on the feasibility, conduct and success of a trial.

The India-based trial management organization initially approached a mix of government and private-sector hospitals with oncology units, proven clinical investigators, required infrastructure and access to a significant patient pool. The results of the initial feasibility analysis demonstrate the impact of various factors on the recruitment funnel.

First-Round Feasibility Results

Institution type:	Public and private
Enrollment period:	10 months
Sites:	7
Patients per month:	+500 (all sites)
Est. total enrollment:	180–200
Enrollment per site per month:	18–20

The sponsor was greatly encouraged by the initial results of the feasibility analysis and began aggressive plans to take the study forward. As part of this planning, it furnished the trial management organization with the full study protocol and scheduled a visit from its Europe-based clinical trial manager to visit and evaluate sites. Upon reviewing the full protocol and complete eligibility criteria, the following challenges became apparent. Among other challenging criteria, the full protocol included the following details:

Figure 5: Patient funnel

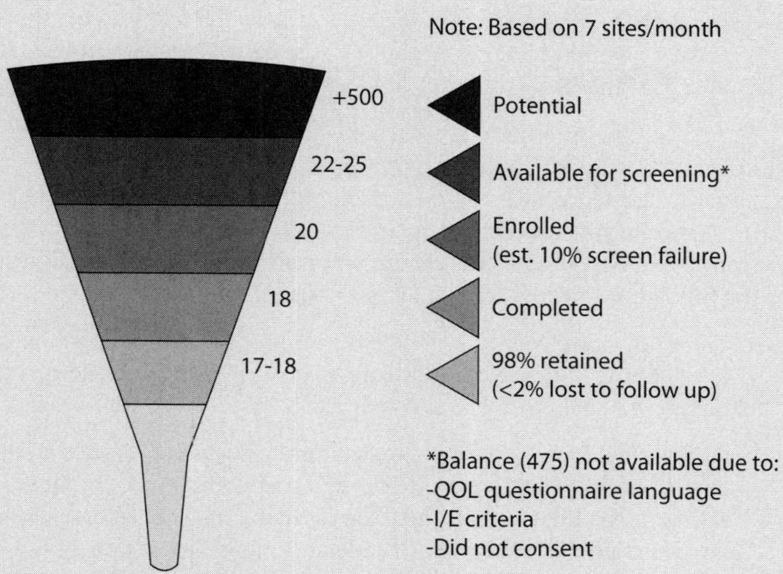

Source: Excel Life Sciences 2010 case study from Phase III Ovarian Cancer study feasibility analysis conducted on behalf of Asia-Pacific based biopharmaceutical company

- Study required patients who had completed at least second-line chemotherapy treatments and were platinum-resistant.
- Drug storage, transportation and accountability issues included strict cold-chain requirements. Specifically, patients would be required to take the study drug home following visits and take one capsule per day all week. The study drug had to remain at the proper temperature during transport to the patient's home and during storage at the home prior to use.
- Requirements included completion of a specialized quality-of-life questionnaire.

These criteria and requirements created significant challenges, because each would have a direct impact on the pool of available patients and study logistics for several reasons specific to emerging markets, such as India, including:

1. The requirement of patients who have completed at least second-line chemotherapy creates challenges in India because, although there is a large population of ovarian cancer patients, only a small portion of those patients receive proper screening, detection, diagnosis and treatment. Furthermore, an even smaller amount proceed through several lines of treatment, either through poor identification or due to

the high cost of chemotherapy treatment. Even though care is generally free of cost at government hospitals in India, the government does charge for chemotherapy treatments, albeit at a lower cost than in private hospitals. For many patients, the cost is too high to pursue further treatment.

2. The requirement to maintain the cold chain of the study drug, not only at the study site but also in transport to and storage at the patient's residence, also results in challenges that affect enrollment figures. Specifically, the temperature average across the country can range from 60 to 100 degrees Fahrenheit. To avoid violation of the cold chain the following considerations had to be made:

    a. The study drug would need to be transported from the site to the patient's home in special temperature-maintaining coolers (thermocol boxes) that include digital thermometers.

    b. Patients would need refrigerators at their residences to store the study drug under the proper conditions. The trial management organization found this would be an issue for many patients who would be seen at public government-funded hospitals, since many of the communities surrounding these centers were on the lower end of the socio-economic scale.

    c. To ensure compliance with the cold chain requirement, the trial management organization would send social workers to patients' homes on a regular basis to log temperature readings.

In addition to these challenges, the trial manager from the sponsor had never before traveled to India and was naïve to some of the unique sensory elements of daily life and unfamiliar with the range of research center settings. During her visit to the country, she toured several state-of-the-art private research clinics and large public government hospitals. The private institutions had a familiar feel to her in that they looked like clinics found in more mature research markets such as Europe and North America. By contrast, the government centers were big, noisy institutions with large numbers of patients.

Interestingly, the government-funded centers are filled with some of the country's top research talent and have performed hundreds of successful local and global studies, including those that were part of USFDA and EMA INDs and NDA submissions. Also, patients visiting government hospitals are eligible for free treatment as part of the country's social healthcare setting and, therefore, those institutions receive a much higher volume of patients. As a result, the initial feasibility analysis included a signficant number of the total estimated enrollment being driven by patients coming from these centers.

Ultimately, when considering the socio-economic challenges that arose from consideration of the public government-funded hospitals and the inaccurate yet understandable concerns of the sponsor related to the aesthetics of those centers, the decision was made to conduct the study only at private hospitals. This decision had a profound impact on study enrollment projections and highlighted some of the elements that must be considered prior to conducting a trial in India or other emerging markets.

Second-Round Feasibility Results

Institution type:	Private only
Enrollment period:	9 months
Phase:	III
Countries:	7 including India
Sites:	7–8 in India
Patients per month:	95–100
Est. enrollment:	60–70
Enrollment per site per month:	7 patients

The second phase of the feasibility, conducted this time only at private research centers, resulted in a reduced total enrollment projection of nearly 200% and a reduction in per site, per month enrollment of 11, from 18 in the feasibility that included government centers to seven in the feasibility including only private centers. Figure 6 contains additional suggestions for items that can be useful in ensuring the placement of the right studies in India and selection of the correct sites.

Patient Retention in a Challenging Study Population

Scenario:

Sponsor:	U.S.-based biopharma
Phase:	II
Condition:	Type 1 Diabetes
Countries:	6 (including India)
Sites:	15 in India
Enrollment:	150 patients (500 globally)

Challenge

Slow enrollment and high turnover prior to engagement of local site management organization (SMO). Patient population included wide age group including adult, adolescent and pediatric patients. Due to length of study, patient's life situations evolved and their ability and desire to stay in the study was challenged.

The SMO visited the sites to evaluate the situation and was hired to manage 15 of a total of 18 sites in India. The company completed a patient seg-

Figure 6: Additional feasibility tips

A face-to-face, on-site visit may be required:

- Gather proper physician buy-in, feedback and establish mutual trust
- Conduct a visual inspection of the facility
- Interview key clinical trial personnel
- Track down answers that may require input from other departments

True "on the ground" local expertise is required:

- Geography
- Transportation routes and access points
- Languages spoken
- Religious and cultural considerations (holidays, views on medicine, etc.)
- Familiarity with hospital and PI experience and reputation
- Willingness of PIs to refer patents

- Disease prevalance (total cases)
- Disease incidence (new cases per year)
- Comparison of prevalence and incidence vs. other known markets
- Typical presentation of disease
- Standard of care
- Number of competing clinical trials taking place for condition in country
  - Number of centers involved in those trials
  - Location of centers involved in those trials
- Number of sites for TA across country
- Number of investigators for specialty across country
- Number of investigators by city Tier (i.e. Tier 1, 2, ...)

Source: The Importance of a Strong Study Feasibility Process, Accurate Site Selection and Patient Enrollment Strategy in India. S Das, Director of Operations and Country Head, Excel Life Sciences at the "ACRP 2009 Global Conference and Exhibition" Denver, CO, April 2009

mentation analysis, analyzing life situations and motivations for each patient type and developing specific strategies and contingency plans:

Retention risks

- 62% of patients lived more than 200 kilometers from the study site
- Relocation due to employment
- Relocation due to college enrollment

- **Females:**
  - Timelines to get married
  - Pregnancy
  - College enrollment
  - Self/parents'/husband's relocation

Figure 7: Case study, volunteers by age group

Percentages of all patients in the study

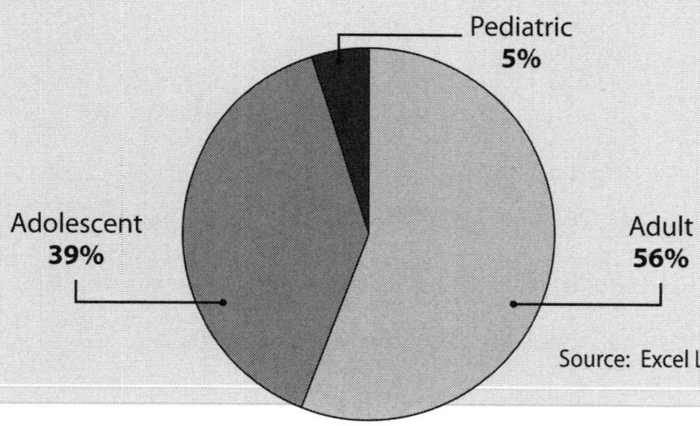

Source: Excel Life Sciences

Solutions

- Placement of highly trained clinical research coordinator at each site to ensure strong day-to-day patient support and follow-up
- Relocation risk:
  - To retain patients for a long run in the study, SMO identified whether the study volunteer could continue participation in the study at another site closer to his or her new residence
  - Offered patients special travel package if they have moved to an area in which no study sites exist (travel, boarding and lodging)
  - **Unique India-centric strategy:** SMO captured information on the hometown/place of origin of study subjects and current location of their parents. Patients in lower/middle income group who have moved from their native homes are likely to return should they be forced to relocate (i.e. in the event of job loss)
  - SMO also captured the school/college addresses and other relevant details for pediatric/adolescent patients
- Other retention activities conducted:
  - Letters to parents of patients in school to update contact details

- Specific email ID at ELS for patients/parents to correspond
- Annual incentives for continuation
- Promote patients as ambassadors/spokespersons in different parts of the country
- Organize regional get-togethers twice a year
- Sponsor recognition of the most active participant
- Sponsor organization of global competition among patients
- Highlight patients who have overcome obstacles to continue the study (distance/relocation/marriage)

Results

- 99% retention of patients in India versus industry average of 75%
- 80% fewer queries than sites in ROW
- **Compliance:** +30,000 visits over course of study
  - 76% of visits happened on actual scheduled visit dates
  - 22% of visits happened within window period
  - 1.67% of visits happened outside of window period
  - 0.43% of visits missed

Author Biography

Dan McDonald is Senior Vice President, Business Strategy, for Excel Life Sciences, a U.S.-based trial management company with a strong focus on supporting trials in India, Europe and the U.S. He has more than 14 years of experience assisting biopharmaceutical companies with patient recruitment, site selection and global clinical research strategies. Previously, Dan served as Senior Vice President of Strategic Development for D. Anderson & Company. He spent nine years at CenterWatch, most recently as General Manager. He also had organizational responsibility for NEIRB, an independent institutional review board. Dan has given over 50 presentations at industry conferences and meetings, plus workshops and sessions on patient recruitment, and has authored chapters in several books on patient recruitment and clinical trial registration.

CHAPTER NINETEEN

The Changing Face of Phase I Recruiting

By Diana L. Anderson-Foster, Ph.D. and Sara Monday

The phase I process is expanding beyond its traditional roots as a first-in-human series of tests in healthy volunteers to a broader scope that includes non-healthy volunteers, trials designed as phase I/phase IIa proof-of-concept studies and drugs tested for combination use.[1] With this transition, phase I studies are becoming more complex, the number of unique procedures per protocol is on the rise, there are more protocol amendments and the associated work burden is escalating. This changing landscape has implications for how subjects can be successfully recruited, enrolled and retained in phase I clinical trials.[2]

Experiencing the new challenges in phase I recruiting first hand are investigative sites and CROs that devise strategies to attract both healthy and non-healthy volunteers into what are widely acknowledged as studies focused on product safety. For the most part, phase I clinical trials still are recruiting healthy volunteers, but there is a distinct trend toward including non-healthy subjects from the outset, as biopharmaceutical companies seek to compress clinical trial timelines, limit costs and look for earlier evidence of safety and efficacy.

This trend signals growth in the search for non-healthy volunteers in phase I research, but also a continuing, if somewhat flat, market for healthy volunteers. As a result, CROs and investigative sites recruiting for these studies may engage different strategies to identify and attract both types of volunteers.

This chapter takes a look at how phase I is changing, how a major CRO and two investigative sites are adapting their practices to reach out to populations needed to participate in this early segment of the research process and the anticipated role of social media in boosting enrollment.

The Changing Phase I Landscape

Phase I is defined as a series of first-in-human short studies in small groups of volunteers, testing for safety and tolerability, pharmacokinetics, single-dose toxicity, food interaction and other critical factors. With revenues grow-

Figure 1: Statement from *Strategic Priorities 2011-2015*

"New challenges posed by globalization, out-sourcing, and increasingly large, multi-facility clinical trials require FDA to refocus its drug review process into one that enables full product life cycle review..."

Source: FDA

ing in the low double digits annually,[3] this phase is set apart because it typically involves overnight stays for healthy volunteers. Increasingly, however, that is changing, as tests are not always being conducted in healthy volunteers and may not follow the classic linear paradigm of phase I followed by phase II and phase III. Rather, proof-of-concept phase I/phase IIa studies are becoming more commonplace as sponsors look to accelerate the clinical trial timeline by collecting phase II-style efficacy information as early as possible.

These changes notwithstanding, the emphasis of phase I still rests firmly on determining the safety of the product being studied. In recent years, the focus on safety has become more intense due to regulatory pressures to improve product safety, starting with earlier identification of safety signals. The FDA, for example, put a final rule into effect in March 2011 that clarifies what safety information must be reported during clinical trials of investigational drugs and biologics.[4] It applies to all trials conducted under an investigational new drug application (IND) or as part of a generic drug application. The new rule requires certain safety information that previously had not been required to be reported to FDA must now be reported within 15 days of becoming aware of an occurrence. There are some specific phase I applications, such as the requirement to report serious adverse events from bioavailability and bioequivalence studies, that are exempt from IND requirements. The agency also put forth *Strategic Priorities 2011-2015*, which spells out how the agency intends to comply with mandates to improve oversight of product safety in an era of increasing globalization and greater outsourcing of study conduct.[5]

Similarly, in Europe, the European Medicines Agency (EMA) launched new pharmacovigilance legislation in December 2010 to improve safety procedures by harmonizing efforts among its Member States.[6,7] Effective July 2012, this legislation as well as regulations from other agencies are requesting risk/benefit assessments from the beginning of the product life cycle, indicating that safety and efficacy must be studied together to produce this data, which begins in phase I.[8]

Complying with these new requirements may mean dosing the targeted population early on, offering the advantage of evaluating safety, efficacy and toxicity sooner. This is particularly valuable in therapeutic areas such as cancer, HIV and infectious disease, in which new compounds might be toxic to healthy volunteers, raising ethical questions about dosing them if they are likely to experience challenging adverse events.

As the phase I picture evolves toward greater safety, it is not surprising that the amount of testing needed to achieve this goal is on the upswing. Research

Figure 2: Increases in procedures per protocol

Procedures and work burden	Phase I	Phase II	Phase III	Phase IV
Unique procedures 2000 – 2003	22.4	21.6	20.0	16.2
Unique procedures 2004 – 2007	30.3	29.2	28.4	26.4
Change in unique procedures	**35.3%**	**35.2%**	**42.0%**	**63.0%**
Total procedures 2000 – 2003	144.7	117.1	93.6	59.1
Total procedures 2004 - 2007	221.8	156.3	147.5	93.9
Change in total procedures	**53.3%**	**33.5%**	**57.6%**	**58.8%**
Total work burden 2000 - 2003	34.3	32.7	27.0	17.9
Total work burden 2004 – 2007	58.4	43.4	43.1	28.4
Change in total work burden	**70.3%**	**32.7%**	**59.7%**	**58.4%**

Note: Values represent means;
Work burden equals time and effort required to complete procedures

Source: Tufts CSDD, <csdd.tufts.edu>, 2011

from the Tufts Center for the Study of Drug Development (CSDD) indicates that the number of procedures per protocol in phase I is larger than that in other phases, having jumped 53.3% in the 2004-2007 time period compared to the 2000-2003 time period.[9] The work burden, a measure of the time and effort needed to complete the procedures, grew a hefty 70.3% over these two time periods, higher than the other phases of clinical research.

Ken Getz, Senior Research Fellow at the Center for the Study of Drug Development, Tufts University School of Medicine and founder and board chair, CISCRP, confirmed that the growing complexity of phase I is linked to the ongoing push toward better safety information. "We are seeing a lot more safety investment activity conducted in phase I. In our research, we see rapid growth in the number of unique procedures, much of which is in response to regulatory pressures to ensure that sponsors are collecting the appropriate safety measures."

Getz said the increase in safety assessments and other activities now being conducted in phase I are part of many companies' efforts to do more at this early stage to avoid having to carry less promising compounds into later phases, for which research becomes much more costly.

Figure 3: Mean number of amendments and changes per amendment by phase

	Phase I	Phase II	Phase III	Phase IIIb/IV
Number of amendments	1.9	2.7	3.5	2.6
Protocol changes per amendment	5.6	6.8	8.5	8.3

Note: Includes only completed protocols (past final database lock) with at least one amendment
Source: Tufts CSDD, <csdd.tufts.edu>, 2011

To complicate matters further, the number of protocol amendments is on the rise, a process that can be quite disruptive to study conduct, particularly in the short studies that typify phase I. Another Tufts CSDD project, this one examining protocol amendments, involved data submitted by 16 biopharmaceutical companies.[10] Results showed that in 1,640 phase I protocols, each protocol averaged 1.9 amendments, generating a mean of 5.6 protocol changes per amendment. More than half of the amendments were completed prior to patient enrollment, but the remaining ones occurred after the studies were underway. All of these changes have an impact on the ease of conducting phase I trials.

Phase I Recruiting: Challenges and Profiles

As a dynamic part of clinical research, phase I is playing a more visible role. The landscape is shifting, so finding the requisite number of healthy and nonhealthy subjects to fulfill phase I studies can be a tall order for sites charged with recruitment, enrollment and retention. This feeds into the larger challenge of finding subjects to participate in all phases of clinical research, an issue that remains one of the biopharmaceutical and medical device industries' most intractable difficulties. Site surveys continue to peg patient recruitment as a major cause of study delays, with data indicating that more than 70% of sites are at least one month behind in enrollment.[11]

Compounding the recruitment dilemma is decreasing public receptivity toward participating in clinical trials. In *Recapturing the Vision*, PricewaterhouseCoopers' Health Research Institute's survey of pharmaceutical stakeholders and consumers details some less than flattering opinions of the industry.[12] The report highlights the limited knowledge many consumers have about the costs and risks of product development. And since many consumers may know even less about the clinical trial process, it is understandable they may view participation as risky, especially if the studies are phase I first-in-human trials.

Phase I has always been set apart, because it usually involves healthy volunteers who typically are confined to an in-patient setting for short periods of time and gain no therapeutic benefit. So prevailing wisdom has been that they must be encouraged to participate through compensation or be motivated to make a meaningful contribution to medical science. They also must have the time and willingness for overnight stays.

To address the range of phase I recruitment challenges, a number of pharmaceutical companies and sites have set up dedicated facilities, expanding the phase I footprint beyond the traditional in-patient units based at academic medical centers.

Covance

Covance, a global CRO, has established a strong presence in the phase I marketplace, starting with its first facility in Madison, Wisc., in 1974. The company has since grown its phase I capability to a total of seven facilities: five in the US, one in Leeds, England, and one in Basel, Switzerland. In total, these facilities house 460 beds, employ more than 500 and offer an array of phase I services, including study conduct and study management.

Figure 4: Covance phase I units

United States	
• Madison, Wisconsin	72 beds
• Evansville, Indiana	80 beds
• Dallas, Texas	80 beds
• Honolulu, Hawaii	50 beds
• Daytona Beach, Florida	64 beds
Europe	
• Leeds, England	72 beds
• Basel, Switzerland	50 beds

Source: Covance 2011

Launa Mitchell, senior director of global clinical operations at Covance, said phase I trials are focusing ever more intensely on safety, and there has been a spike in combined phase I/phase IIa proof-of-concept studies. With protocols reflecting this changing phase I paradigm, studies are seeking subjects who fall into three buckets: normal, healthy volunteers; special populations; and patient populations. Special populations are loosely defined as those who have high cholesterol, high blood pressure, obesity or other specific health conditions, or belong to ethnic groups such as Japanese or African-American, but do not have the disease being studied.

For the most part, methods for phase I recruitment remain fairly typical, such as television, radio, newspapers, medical screenings at shopping malls and, more recently, social media, because the large majority of studies Covance conducts are seeking normal, healthy volunteers. "We aren't fully into patients yet in phase I. In the protocols, we're seeing approximately 80% healthy volunteers, 10% from special populations and 10% with the disease," said Mitchell. Protocols sometimes have multiple arms that include subjects from some or all of these groups.

Importantly, Mitchell pointed out that this ratio is not static—the trend is toward greater inclusion of patients with the disease. "We are being asked more and more to get patients into the phase I space," she said.

Besides its standard recruiting practices, Covance uses two particularly successful strategies. First is "warm calling," which refers to outbound calls from the company's database; and second is the Refer-A-Friend program. In this program, subjects who have participated can refer friends or family who are not in the database, and if they meet the screening criteria the referring individual receives $200.

Covance also operates three live call centers—one for the U.S. and two others embedded in the U.K. and Basel sites. The call centers screen individuals who respond to advertising for specific studies and answer individuals' questions about enrolling in Covance studies.

For studies seeking non-healthy subjects, the company relies heavily on its relationships with physicians who treat the patients needed for upcoming or ongoing studies. "We are looking to the physicians to help us find this population, as this is new ground for us in phase I," said Mitchell. "We are also educating doctors about the phase I space. To build this relationship, we do a lot of face-to-face interaction, and it's important to consider what's in it for the doctor." Fortunately, many investigators are already familiar with Covance from their work in later-phase studies.

The company hires physicians as both full-time and part-time principal investigators in its phase I clinics. Covance does not recruit from those investigators' practices, but the investigators can use their relationships to inform other physicians about ongoing studies.

These comprehensive recruitment strategies are paying off, as Mitchell said the dropout rate in phase I is less than 3%. "We try to get volunteers involved in activities, offer free Internet service, a pool table and a quiet area," she said. "The few volunteers who drop out generally do so because of a family emergency or a personal situation."

Metroplex Clinical Research Center (MCRC)

MCRC, a large investigative site in Dallas, Texas, conducts studies in a variety of therapeutic indications, but its phase I work is focused largely on autoimmune diseases, particularly rheumatoid arthritis (RA). One of the medical directors, Dr. Roy M. Fleischmann, said he has seen an approximate 20%-25% increase in the amount of phase I work at the site recently. "There are probably 30 drugs in development now," he said.

Most are seeking healthy volunteers, but with the uptick in phase I studies, more are targeting patients with disease. This is expected to increase as clinical studies begin in biosimilars, large, complex biologic therapies sometimes used to treat patients suffering from autoimmune disorders and cancer. Biosimilars may not be well tolerated by healthy volunteers, so it is likely that upcoming phase I studies will seek non-healthy subjects.

There is strong interest in biosimilars, for which an abbreviated regulatory pathway is just starting to be defined by the FDA. In February 2012, the agency released three draft guidances on the subject.[13, 14, 15] Chad Fragle, CEO of

MCRC, said, "We have been approached by a number of companies looking to conduct biosimilar studies in our areas of expertise, and we expect interest in this area to grow as the regulatory pathway is better defined."

With this flurry of activity, MCRC's medical directors, who also are private practice rheumatologists, are able to recruit many subjects from internal sources, including separate databases of RA, lupus, scleroderma and dermatology patients. With RA studies in particular, upwards of 80% of subjects routinely are recruited from the database. In addition, notices in the private practice waiting room announce upcoming studies, and the staff conducts chart reviews. Generally, the site finds the best subjects are those who already are patients of the private practice. To complement the database effort, the site frequently advertises in print media, as well as television and radio. With more patients using the internet, MCRC also posts current studies on the company web site and at www.clinicalconnection.com.

When MCRC entered the phase I market in 2007, the site started with two beds. In March 2011, it opened a secured unit with 12 beds in 3,500 square feet. Most stays last one to three nights. The space is a hotel-like environment and includes a recreational facility, free WiFi and dining facilities providing meals that may be study-specific.

Regarding retention, Fragle said the site places a heavy emphasis on good customer service, "but our biggest strength is that this is a niche practice of chronic care patients. We have developed a long-term relationship with them, which helps with retention."

Profil Institute for Clinical Research

Profil Institute for Clinical Research in San Diego is a private site dedicated solely to the conduct of early clinical trials, exclusively in diabetes and obesity, ranging from first-in-man to phase IIa proof-of-concept studies. Approximately one-third of the study population includes healthy volunteers, and the remaining two-thirds have the targeted disease. Dennis DeRosia, director of business development, said the volume of phase I and combination phaseI/phase IIa studies conducted at the site are definitely on the rise, fueled by the global diabetes epidemic. He said from 2005 to 2009, revenues grew 20% annually.

To recruit the desired number of non-healthy subjects, Profil maintains a database stratified by Type 1 and Type 2 diabetics, ethnic groups, HbA1c categories, co-morbidities and concomitant medications. In addition, the site works very closely with the American Diabetes Association (ADA) and the Juvenile Diabetes Research Foundation (JDRF) in San Diego. "We attend all of their functions, such as bicycle rides and walks, and find that people are curious about what's being tested. It's a fruitful way to recruit. Also, we've educated diabetes educators about our studies and even had the national president of ADA visit our facility in recognition of our contributions," said DeRosia.

Aside from these tactics designed to attract a specialized population, Profil utilizes standard recruitment practices such as television and radio advertising, local shopper ads mailed to homes, the newspaper and e-mail blasts to bring in new patients as well as normal, healthy volunteers. Subjects in the database may receive phone calls to advise them of upcoming studies, and to encourage retention the site makes reminder calls to patients participating in outpatient portions of studies.

According to DeRosia, diabetic patients are often highly motivated to participate because of the desire to help others in the diabetic community. "Only the diabetic can help us find the answer," he said.

The site has 35 beds and more than 160 employees in 28,000 square feet. Six beds are dedicated to clamp studies, which DeRosia explains is a rare offering. "Increasingly, FDA and EMA like to see early clamp data from investigational compounds to get a sense of safety and efficacy," he said. (A clamp study is a procedure that evaluates the blood glucose-lowering action of antidiabetic agents and determines their time action profile. The technique provides reliable quantitative data needed for a complete characterization of a new diabetes drug.)

Social Media in Phase I

With the internet practically ubiquitous in developed countries, and social media sites such as Facebook, Twitter and MySpace entrenched as commonplace in the daily lives of millions across the globe, it is logical to explore whether these tools can prove valuable as avenues for phase I patient recruitment and retention activities. Because social media are still a relatively new phenomenon, they are in early stages of consideration for their recruitment and retention potential, but going forward this is destined to change with increased understanding of their impact and as they become standard tools for information sharing.

Anticipated growth in the use of social media is likely to mirror the heavy use of the internet by people researching information on health care and disease conditions. *The Social Life of Health Information, 2011*, a report from the Pew Research Center's Internet & American Life Project, provides a wealth of information documenting this trend.[16] Of particular note is that in the U.S., 59% of all adults have looked online for information on health topics, such as disease or treatment, and 25% of adults have read someone else's commentary or experience about health or medical issues on an online news group, web site, or blog. Internet users with chronic conditions show even greater use, and among wireless users, who outpace traditional internet users in virtually all measures of online searches for health information, 37% reported reading about others' health experiences.

Regarding social media, the Pew report states that as of September 2010, 62% of adult internet users claim to be using a social network site such as MySpace or Facebook. Of that group, 15% sought health information and 11% posted comments, queries or information about health or medical matters.

Figure 5: Some statistics on the use of the internet and social media

- 59% of all adults have looked online for information on health topics, such as disease or treatment
- 25% of adults have read some else's commentary or experience about health or medical issues on an online news group, web site, or blog
- 19% of adults have watched an online video about health or medical issues
- 18% of adults have consulted online reviews of particular drugs or medical treatments
- Of those who use social networking sites, 7% of adults have received health information from those sites
- Of those who use social networking sites, 5% of adults have posted comments, queries or information about health or medical matters

Source: The Social Life of Health Information, 2011

These are powerful trends, especially when backed by data that of the 800 million Facebook users across the world in 2011,[17] 350 million of them are accessing Facebook via mobile devices; and of the 100 million Twitter users, 50% post daily.[18] But applying this trend to phase I patient recruitment strategies is an evolving story. In particular, the interactive nature of social media sites can raise concerns for companies looking to recruit subjects, as it is not clear how companies should respond to posted comments. Does the individual want to voice an opinion about a potential drug or class of drugs, report an adverse event or lodge a complaint? Companies are rightfully concerned about how to handle this information, particularly adverse events, which must be reported. But because there are so many unknowns linked to these postings, such as whether the information meets the standard for an adverse event or a serious adverse event,[19] companies are likely to sidestep this problem by directing visitors to web sites that list clinical trial information but do not allow them to post comments.

The industry has been anticipating direction from the FDA as to how to handle these issues, and in December 2011, the FDA released its first draft guidance on suggested ways for life sciences companies to respond to statements and requests for information made through social media by individuals.[20] This is the first of several anticipated social media guidances from the agency.

The three companies profiled, Covance, MCRC and Profil Institute, have phase I studies listed on their respective web sites, but all are in early stages of utilizing social media for recruitment purposes. Launa Mitchell of Covance says her company is using Facebook, mobile text messaging and Twitter. The Facebook page refers visitors to www.testwiththebest.com, Covance's web site for phase I patient recruitment. In addition, the company is developing a mobile phone app for patient recruitment under the name of testwiththebest.

At Profil, the site is just beginning to consider social media. The company has yet to implement mobile text messaging but has set up a Facebook page with basic information about Profil. No studies are listed on the Facebook page, but it does contain links to the American Diabetes Association and the Juvenile Diabetes Research Foundation. Dennis DeRosia explained, "We remain very conservative concerning our social media outreach, mainly because of regulatory issues. On our web site, we remain in control of the information and everything there that reaches out to potential volunteers is pre-approved by an IRB. On Facebook, we can't control what people post and, therefore, remain guarded."

At MCRC, the company is experiencing a high volume of hits on its Web site and utilizes www.clinicalconnection to list ongoing studies. Similar to Profil, the company has established a Facebook page, which provides basic facts about the site but no study-specific information.

Definitely Dynamic

All of clinical research is undergoing a transformation related to rigid timelines, budgetary constraints and a greater emphasis on product safety. Leading the pack is phase I, a previously quiet, somewhat behind-the-scenes part of clinical research that is now emerging as a highly visible driving force, designed to sniff out promising compounds from laggards from the beginning. To bolster this effort, the number of procedures is rising, which generates more data sooner, including an earlier look at safety signals and efficacy. Chad Fragle of MCRC said, "The level of detail associated with phase I has definitely increased in terms of more procedures and very strict timeframes for drawing labs. All of this is designed to learn more about a compound earlier."

With a continuing shift toward more phase I work, the need for more non-healthy subjects is increasing, as evidenced by the already changing ratio of healthy to non-healthy volunteers being recruited to fill new studies. To satisfy this demand, the array of techniques used to recruit and retain subjects will be modified to reflect the relatively new phenomenon of enrolling non-healthy subjects in phase I studies. For the most part, traditional methods will continue, such as radio, television, newspaper, phone calls and e-mail blasts, but as technology evolves and more people receive information via wireless mobile devices, they will be supplemented by greater use of social media. As this happens, companies must position themselves to respond, in keeping with new guidelines.

Overall, as phase I studies become more complex to satisfy the greater emphasis on safety, more resources and attention will be directed toward recruiting and retaining subjects for this part of the clinical development timeline.

Author Biographies

Over a career spanning more than 25 years, Diana L. Anderson-Foster, Ph.D., has helped pioneer best practices in patient recruitment and retention for global clinical trials—first as founder, president and CEO of D. Anderson & Company and today as president of DAC Patient Recruitment Services, an Imperial company. Her book credits include *International Patient Recruitment: Regulatory Guidelines, Customs and Practices*; *A Guide to Patient Recruitment*; and *A Guide to Patient Recruitment and Retention*. In 2006, *PharmaVOICE* named her among the 100 Most Inspiring People in the Life Sciences Industry. She also received an International Women of Influence Award from the Global EXEC Women's International Council in 2008, among other honors.

Sara Monday is Chief Operating Officer for Metroplex Clinical Research Center in Dallas, Texas, a Rheumatology Research Site. Previously, she was a site manager for a national SMO and co-founder of a Trials Management Organization. Sara has served as chair, co-chair and treasurer of the Site Managers Forum, as well as president of her local ACRP chapter, and has been active as a speaker for ACRP and as contributing author for the Monitor. She also served on the Government Affairs Committee for ACRP in 2005 and 2006.

References

1. Guidance for Industry Codevelopment of two or more unmarketed investigational drugs for use in combination. Draft Guidance. Food and Drug Administration. Center for Drug Evaluation and Research. December 2010. www.fda.gov/downloads/Drugs/Guidance ComplianceRegulatoryInformation/Guidances/UCM236669.pdf, accessed December 14, 2011.

2. Rosenberg, R. *Trend shifts away from phase I 'healthy volunteers.'* CWWeekly. May 16, 2011. www.centerwatch.com/news-online/article/1625/trend-shifts-away-from-phase-i-healthy-volunteers, accessed December 9, 2011.

3. *The Phase I clinical study market: A 2007 assessment.* Thomson CenterWatch, January 2007.

4. Safety reporting requirements for INDs and BA/BE studies. Guidance for industry and investigators. Food and Drug Administration. September 2010. www.fda.gov/downloads/Drugs/Guidance ComplianceRegulatoryInformation/Guidances/UCM227351.pdf, accessed December 11, 2011.

5. Strategic priorities. Responding to the public health challenges of the 21st century. Food and Drug Administration. www.fda.gov/downloads/aboutfda/reportsmanualsforms/reports/ucm252128.pdf, accessed December 8, 2011.

6. Directive 2010/84/EU of the European Parliament and of the Council of 15 December 2010. http://ec.europa.eu/health/files/eudralex/vol-1/dir_2010_84/dir_2010_84_en.pdf, accessed December 8, 2011.

7. Regulation (EU) No 1235/2010 of the European Parliament and of the Council of 15 December 2010, http://ec.europa.eu/health/files/eudralex/vol-1/reg_2010_1235/reg_2010_1235_en.pdf, accessed December 8, 2011.

8. Shah, K. *Fixing the failure rate.* Next Generation Pharmaceuticals. May 13, 2010. http://issuu.com/gdsdigital/docs/ngpus18, accessed December 8, 2011.

9. Getz, K.A., Campo, R.A., Kaitin, K.I. *Variability in protocol design complexity by phase and therapeutic area.* Drug Information Journal. 2011(45): 413-20.

10. Getz, K.A., Zuckerman, R., Cropp, A.B., et al. *Measuring the incidence, causes, and repercussions of protocol amendments.* Drug Information Journal. 2011(45): 265-75.

11. CenterWatch Survey of Investigative Sites in the US: 2009

12. Farino, A.L., Claude, P.J., Riewerts, B., et al. *Recapturing the vision: Restoring trust in the pharmaceutical industry by translating expectations into actions.* PricewaterhouseCoopers' Health Research Institute. 2006. www.pwc.com/he_IL/il/publications/assets/11recapturing.pdf, accessed December 10, 2011.

13. Scientific considerations to demonstrating biosimilarity to a reference product. Draft Guidance. Food and Drug Administration. February 2012. www.fda.gov/downloads/Drugs/GuidanceCompliance RegulatoryInformation/Guidances/UCM291128.pdf, accessed February 12, 2012.

14. Quality considerations in demonstrating biosimilarity to a reference protein product. Draft Guidance. Food and Drug Administration. February 2012. www.fda.gov/downloads/Drugs/Guidance ComplianceRegulatoryInformation/Guidances/UCM291134.pdf, accessed February 12, 2012.

15. Biosimilars: Questions and Answers Regarding Implementation of the Biologics Price Competition and Innovation Act of 2009. Draft Guidance. Food and Drug Administration. February 2012. www.fda.gov/downloads/Drugs/GuidanceComplianceRegulatoryInformation/Guidances/UCM273001.pdf, accessed February 12, 2012.

16. Fox, S. *The Social life of health information, 2011.* Pew Research Center's Internet & American Life Project, May 2011. www.pewInternet.org/~/media//Files/Reports/2011/PIP_Social_Life_of_Health_Info.pdf, accessed December 13, 2011.

17. Statistics. Facebook, December 2011. www.facebook.com/press/info.php?statistics, accessed December 13, 2011.

18. Hachman, M. Twitter continues to soar in popularity, site's numbers reveal. Pcmag.com, September 8, 2011. www.pcmag.com/article2/0,2817,2392658,00.asp, accessed December 13, 2011.

19. Neuer A. Facebook and pharma – an uneasy alliance. ECliniqua. September 19, 2011. www.bio-itworld.com/2011/09/19/facebook-pharma-uneasy-alliance.html, accessed January 10, 2012.

20. Guidance for Industry, Responding to Unsolicited Requests for Off-Label Information About Prescription Drugs and Medical Devices. Draft Guidance. Food and Drug Administration. December 2011. www.fda.gov/downloads/drugs/guidancecomplianceregulatory information/guidances/ucm285145.pdf, accessed January 10, 2012.

CHAPTER TWENTY

The Future of Patient Recruitment and Retention

By Diana L. Anderson-Foster, Ph.D.

In writing the final chapter of this book, it strikes me that much has changed since 1998 when the first edition was published. But perhaps more striking is that much has remained the same in this challenging area of the clinical trials process.

Despite the intensity of the focus on enrollment, statistics show accrual rates continue to decline, particularly in the U.S., Canada and Western Europe. The obstacles to delivering patients to complete clinical trials continue to grow. Protocol complexity has increased dramatically, making patient participation overly demanding and retention extremely difficult. Another particularly significant factor is the churning of investigators and the unanswered question: why do nearly half (45%) of all global investigators quit each year, never to participate in another clinical trial experience? This points to the strong need to better understand how we can support, train and educate investigators and study staff around the world to fully engage and enroll patients into clinical trials.

As experts in the field weigh in, it is more than interesting to try to evaluate and determine what the future may hold and the steps required to ensure higher levels of patient recruitment and retention effectiveness. Tom Ruane, vice president of patient recruitment and retention at Quintiles and a long-time participant in the recruitment arena, believes we must trust in what we know to be successful. Ruane and his team believe there is a critical need to "return to basics and the simplicity of implementing fundamentals that are metrics-driven and form the core of a recruitment and retention platform."

Recent surveys conducted by DAC Patient Recruitment Services among study coordinators corroborate Ruane's assessment. The training needs of study coordinators include learning more about rudimentary recruitment and retention practices and how to measure their effectiveness. Surveys strongly suggest the clinical trials enterprise is focusing too much attention on new and unknown strategies and tactics in the race to enroll and retain subjects in clinical trials. Rudimentary approaches include the need to be culturally sensitive and to leverage the rapport and trust between investigative site staff and their patients.

Steve Swanson, CEO of DAC, said it will be critical in the foreseeable future to develop protocol-specific strategies that minimize risk and optimize accruals. This requires a suite of solutions not readily considered and offered today that involve all stakeholders—including sponsors, CROs and comprehensive recruitment providers—to collaborate actively and effectively. These collaborations must bring robust technology (e.g., social media, electronic health records) together with a clear understanding of the human elements within the study and the working teams. Increasingly, these solutions must seamlessly span both geography and cultures.

"At DAC, we continue to shape the business in the ability to deliver these solutions. In addition, we emphasize working with sites globally in the critical areas of compliance, training and education. Only then can we 'tip the needle' in favor of increasing accrual rates and expediting the recruitment and retention process," said Swanson.

Three Critical Areas of Engagement

Ken Getz, Senior Research Fellow at the Center for the Study of Drug Development, Tufts University School of Medicine and founder and board chair, CISCRP, speaks about three engagement areas as critical and untapped drivers of recruitment and retention success. These three areas require ongoing investment of time and resources, but hold the potential to play a major role in improving accrual and completion rates in the future.

1. **Engaging the public through education and outreach to:** rebuild trust in the clinical research enterprise, help the public draw a personal connection between clinical trials and public health, and teach the public to become informed and proactive future volunteers.
2. **Engaging healthcare providers and healthcare educators (e.g., pharmacists, publishers) to become ambassadors and partners in:** spreading the word about clinical trial activity, making referrals into clinical trials and suggesting resources for patients to turn to for additional information.
3. **Engaging patient and disease advocacy groups as active collaborators and partners in:** setting research agendas, developing feasible and relevant protocols, helping to fund future research studies and drawing participation from their vast patient memberships.

Accountability/Predictability

Patient recruitment has evolved greatly over the past decade. Tactics have expanded well beyond traditional chart review, radio, TV and print to include database driven, targeted direct mail and a host of eRecruitment techniques that capitalize on the continually expanding role of the internet for people seeking healthcare-related information or dialogue.

Rick Malcolm, CEO of Acurian, says one factor that has limited the adoption of these increasingly sophisticated techniques is the historical lack of predictability of the results of various tactical campaigns, and the absence of accountability by the patient recruitment vendor when the tactics are ineffective and fail to affect recruitment and retention performance. Fortunately, he said, recruitment specialists are gaining expertise in more robust and reliable predictive modeling and in adopting higher levels of accountability.

"I fully expect to see a steady increase in the accuracy of predictions/feasibility from the better, more sophisticated recruitment companies. Also I expect to see greater shared financial risk by the recruitment companies as they gain confidence in their predicted results. I would expect these two factors—greater predictability and greater accountability—will support broader use of centralized patient recruitment service providers. This may come at the expense of CRO change orders for more investigative sites and/or more time—the alternative to utilizing a specialty recruitment company," said Malcolm.

The Problem Isn't Going Away

Over the past few years, interest has grown in the potential to improve the site selection process as a primary means to ensure patient recruitment success. Despite sponsor and CRO use of rich, de-identified data (e.g., from prescriber data, patient demographic and psychographic data, insurance claims data, electronic health records data) to identify sites with the highest concentration of patients, recruitment and retention is still at issue. One can use sophisticated techniques to find a watering hole, but one still has to get the horse to drink from it.

Clinical trials continue to run late due in part to poor and ineffective recruitment and retention, and many sites still enroll fewer patients than expected and required. Of course, much of the recruitment and retention challenge increasingly is due to restrictive study volunteer eligibility criteria (i.e., inclusion and exclusion) that dramatically reduce the number of a site's patients who may qualify for a study.

Regardless, eliminating the need for central patient recruitment support by improved site selection, while a desirable goal, isn't going to happen. Rather, increasing protocol complexity coupled with competition for patients from other clinical trials, will have the opposite effect of fueling a need for more centralized patient recruitment support for the foreseeable future.

The future of patient recruitment and retention holds more questions than answers. What role will social media and internet advertising play? How will GCP-ICH regulations guide us? Can we expect increasing or easing regulatory burden? How will the landscape of global investigative sites evolve?

Will we see more patient-centric clinical trials that deliberately cut out site involvement and engage study volunteers directly using online solutions? Will we see advocacy group pairings and funding of research hand in hand with pharmaceutical and biotechnology companies to capture potential participant interest?

There is no question that minority recruitment initiatives will become increasingly important, from both scientific and regulatory perspectives. As clinical research targets more focused patient subgroups, professionals will be required to better understand special populations and how to reach them effectively. The complexities of culture, rituals, language, healthcare access and diverse patient perception speaks to the need for significant research to validate what role recruitment and retention must play among minority communities.

Future trends quite possibly will require us to take a step back and evaluate the processes that ultimately lead us to more measurable, substantive outcome criteria to guide our efforts. They may require us to work more closely with organizations such as the Center for Information and Study on Clinical Research Participation (CISCRP) to help grow the understanding of clinical trials around the globe. If 75% of the U.S. population has never heard of a clinical trial, then what of the other regions of the world where we are heavily becoming more and more reliant on patient participation?

The answers to these questions currently may elude us, but there is no question that this challenging field will continue to become more sophisticated, requiring higher levels of expertise with every passing year. Mistakes can and will be made without the involvement of industry experts. Expertise is essential to protecting the integrity of the science behind clinical trials and improving the lives of those who not only participate in studies but also bring advances in medicine to all.

Reading this book conveys your commitment to and interest in improving patient recruitment and retention success. From China to India to Ukraine to Spain, challenges remain. The solutions rest with the current experts and those to come.

Recently, I met a young lady at a large pharmaceutical company who was new to the recruitment team and a recent graduate of Rutgers University in Princeton, N.J. She had joined the team after working as an intern.

When I asked her why she had chosen a career in such a challenging field, she said, "I know from personal experience that new drug development is dependent on volunteers coming forward to participate in clinical trials. The methodology to recruit and retain volunteers involves so many variables that require many levels of understanding, all directly tied to developing relationships and a better understanding of what is involved in clinical trials."

It seems the science behind clinical research may be the "easy part of the work." What remains is the coordination, compassion and willingness of study teams to engage and believe in new solutions, and implement these solutions.

All of the individuals who contributed to this book are willing and able to take on and continue the cause in the hope we will eventually—one trial at a time, if necessary—move closer to solutions to bring improved quality of life to many.

Author Biography

Over a career spanning more than 25 years, Diana L. Anderson-Foster, Ph.D., has helped pioneer best practices in patient recruitment and retention for global clinical trials—first as founder, president and CEO of D. Anderson & Company and today as president of DAC Patient Recruitment Services, an Imperial company. Her book credits include *International Patient Recruitment: Regulatory Guidelines, Customs and Practices, A Guide to Patient Recruitment* and *A Guide to Patient Recruitment and Retention*. In 2006, *PharmaVOICE* named her among the 100 Most Inspiring People in the Life Sciences Industry. She also received an International Women of Influence Award from the Global EXEC Women's International Council in 2008, among other honors.

ABOUT THE AUTHOR

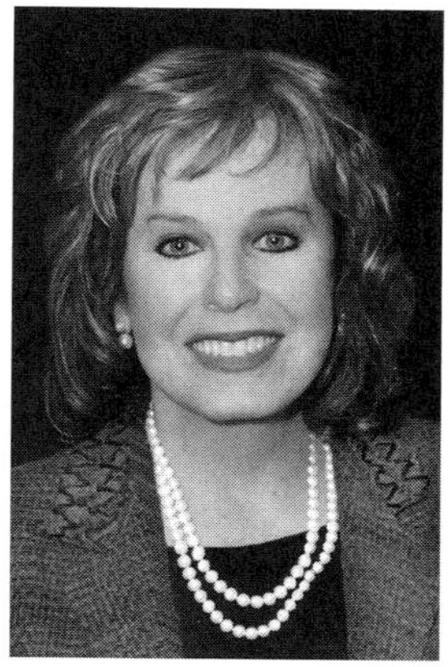

As president of DAC Patient Recruitment Services (formerly D. Anderson & Company), an Imperial company, Dr. Diana L. Anderson-Foster, Ph.D., is an international thought leader in patient recruitment and retention for clinical trials and in the intricacies of site management.

Over the past two decades, she has addressed audiences across five continents, authored hundreds of white papers and presentations and written four authoritative industry books. Her self-published *International Patient Recruitment: Regulatory Guidelines, Customs and Practices* provides an expository view of legislation governing patient recruitment in 23 countries and serves as a teaching tool for several colleges and universities, along with her earlier works *A Guide to Patient Recruitment, A Guide to Patient Recruitment and Retention and 50 Ways to Cope with Arthritis.*

Dr. Anderson-Foster is considered a pioneer in patient recruitment for clinical trials, helping to create and grow the cottage industry into a multibillion-dollar specialty area. She has led DAC through its evolution as a niche site management organization, Rheumatology Research International, to its current status as a premier patient recruitment organization. Her early tenure leading an SMO gives her a unique understanding of how sites operate and what they need to reach enrollment goals within targeted timelines. RRI was one of the first SMOs serving the rheumatology sector and became a model for crafting clinical strategies based on individual site needs. She parlayed that experience into DAC's site-focused recruitment and retention business model, which pairs project managers with sites to customize services and help sites meet short- and long-term goals. She also is part owner of a multi-specialty clinical research site in Dallas that has completed more than 1,000 phase I-IV studies in a variety of therapeutic areas, with a focus on immunology.

Leveraging 20 years of experience in 100 countries, the DAC team offers four phases of consulting services, providing foundational support for clients to build internal recruitment and retention resources and build global metric-supported recruitment and retention success. She designed early curriculum for DAC's Best Recruitment and Retention Practices training programs, which prepared project managers, clinical research associates, coordinators, site directors and investigators to meet recruitment and retention challenges.

In 2009 she was recognized by the Global EXEC Women's International Council as an International Woman of Influence and in 2006 by PharmaVOICE as one of its 100 Most Inspiring People in the Life-Sciences Industry.

Dr. Anderson-Foster currently serves on the boards of the Center for Information & Study on Clinical Research Participation (CISCRP), *Journal for Clinical Studies* and *R&D Directions*. Her memberships include the Patient Recruitment Organization Steering Committee, American College of Rheumatology Research and Education Foundation Development Advisory Council and American Foundation for the Blind Center on Vision Loss Development Committee.

She is past chairman of the board of the Association of Clinical Research Professionals (ACRP) and past president of the Association of Rheumatology Health Professionals (ARHP).

ABOUT CENTERWATCH

Founded in 1994, CenterWatch is a trusted source and global destination of clinical trials information for both professionals and patients. CenterWatch provides a wide variety of information services including grant leads for investigative sites; business development leads for contract service providers; postings of career opportunities; listings of clinical trials actively seeking patients; advertising and promotional opportunities; and proprietary business analysis and data about the global clinical trials industry.

As a pioneer in publishing clinical trials information, CenterWatch was the first web site to publish detailed information about clinical trials that could be freely accessed by patients and their advocates. Today, we have the largest online database of actively recruiting, industry-sponsored clinical trials.

Visit centerwatch.com, call (617) 948-5100 or email customerservice@centerwatch.com for more in-depth information on the wide variety of products and services CenterWatch offers.

CenterWatch Products and Service Offerings

- Periodicals and Business News
- Grant Notification and Site Identification Services
- Market Intelligence Services
- Patient Enrollment Services
- Patient Education
- Career Services
- Clinical Research Training Guides
- Regulatory Compliance
- Medical Writing Services
- Information Solutions and Content Licensing
- Business Development and Partnership Opportunities

Periodicals and Business News

The CenterWatch Monthly

The CenterWatch Monthly, our flagship publication, is a premier industry resource providing in-depth, authoritative business coverage for the clinical trials community, including unparalleled competitive market intelligence and clinical study leads and the most detailed drug pipeline analysis in the industry—all in one comprehensive publication featuring original CenterWatch data.

CWWeekly

CWWeekly is a leading news source providing expanded analysis on the week's top business and financial headlines and trends. Other features include: market intelligence, patient recruitment tips, drug intelligence and clinical study leads.

Research Practitioner

This bi-monthly journal is a valuable, educational and career advancement resource that provides in-depth and practical "how-to" articles about clinical research management trends, ethical and legal principles, regulatory issues and more. Subscribers can earn up to 18 CNE credits per year.

CenterWatch News Online

CenterWatch News Online (centerwatch.com/news-online) is a dynamic and easy-to-navigate online service featuring real-time objective news reports covering timely stories and emerging trends in the global clinical research industry. Features include: breaking news and top headlines as selected by the CenterWatch editorial staff, news beats featuring relevant content on various industry segments and proprietary CenterWatch data.

Grant Notification and Site Identification Services

TrialWatch for Sites

A complimentary grant notification service designed to help research centers easily connect with sponsors and CROs seeking qualified investigators for upcoming or ongoing active trials. Sites complete a brief online profile that is stored in a database and then matched against grant requests from sponsors and CROs. When a match is found, the site information is forwarded to the requesting company for consideration. Site profiles can be completed at centerwatch.com/trialwatch_signup.

TrialWatch for Sponsors and CROs

A complimentary site identification service that helps companies quickly and effectively identify active and qualified investigative sites worldwide to conduct upcoming and active phase I through phase IV clinical trials. Confidential requests can be submitted online at centerwatch.com/clinical-trials/trialwatch.

Research Center Profile Pages

Research Center Profile Pages, located on centerwatch.com, are an easy and cost-effective way for sites to showcase detailed information online about their site offerings and expertise to secure clinical research grants and contracts, increase their site's exposure and reach a captive and targeted audience. Profile Pages are completely customizable and can include images, video presentations, links to company documents, trial listings and more.

Market Intelligence Services

Custom Market Intelligence Services

Unprecedented business knowledge of the clinical research enterprise, combined with proprietary data and global contacts, gives CenterWatch a unique and objective position to perform rich and insightful quantitative and qualitative market intelligence services.

Our comprehensive offerings focus on all aspects of the life sciences and clinical trials industry and include secondary data analysis, interviews, focus group research and a broad range of customer surveys such as outsourcing and vendor evaluations, research and examination of new industry technologies, company performance and relationships, post-trial analysis to gauge site success, volatility of global investigative site infrastructure and more.

Our experienced market research team works directly with companies to provide mission-critical information and detailed market analysis their organizations need to make more effective business decisions. We provide final reports for all commissioned studies and also offer presentations and facilitated discussions.

Clinical Trials Data Library

The *CenterWatch Clinical Trials Data Library* is a valuable online and searchable resource providing access to comprehensive data on the life sciences and clinical research industry. Derived from several industry sources, including proprietary, CenterWatch-conducted surveys, data charts range from analysis of global economic trends and clinical research practices to examinations of partnerships and drug development pipelines and performance. Charts can be conveniently downloaded, copied and pasted into PowerPoint or Word documents to create dynamic, data-driven business reports and conference presentations, prepare strategic marketing, financial and business development plans and study current and historical activity for training and roundtable discussions.

Patient Enrollment Services

Clinical Trials Listing Service™

As one of the first web sites to publish clinical trials actively seeking study volunteers, CenterWatch continues to be a leading resource for patients interested in clinical trial participation receiving more than one million visitors annually to our listings. When companies post a trial on our *Clinical Trials Listing Service™*, now the largest online database of industry-funded global clinical trials, this targeted population has direct access to these listings via a range of distribution channels including: email messaging programs, email alerts for new trial postings, social media efforts, top search engine rankings including Search Clinical Trials, RSS clinical news feeds and collaborative relationships with health associations and other non-profit organizations.

Patient Education

Volunteering for a Clinical Trial

An easy-to-read, IRB-approved pamphlet designed as a quick reference guide for potential volunteers interested in participating in a research study. It includes an overview of the clinical trials process and answers some of the most commonly asked questions about volunteering for a clinical trial. Translations available in Spanish, French, Italian, Portuguese, Dutch and German.

Understanding the Informed Consent Process

A comprehensive, IRB-approved brochure providing study volunteers with important information regarding the informed consent process, including facts and information about the volunteer's "Bill of Rights." Translation available in Spanish.

Career Services

JobWatch

JobWatch (centerwatch.com/jobwatch) is a key clinical research recruitment and career resource for professionals currently involved in the industry or professionals interested in obtaining a career in the life sciences or clinical research field.

JobWatch provides job listings, upcoming industry events, educational programs, company profiles and more. Registered job seekers can also manage resumes, set up email alerts and apply directly for positions online. Employers can review resumes, post and manage current openings and maximize exposure with a variety of recruitment and advertising opportunities online along with utilizing the various distribution channels *JobWatch* offers to reach professionals.

Clinical Research Training Guides

CenterWatch's training guide series offers effective and practical tools for those interested in clinical research as well as seasoned professionals seeking to better understand their roles and improve the management of their clinical trials operations in a safe and ethical manner.

- *Becoming a Successful Clinical Research Investigator*
- *The CRA's Guide to Monitoring Clinical Research*
- *The CRC's Guide to Coordinating Clinical Research*
- *Protecting Study Volunteers in Research* (CME credits)
- *Global Regulatory Systems: A Strategic Primer for Biopharmaceutical Product Development and Registration*

Regulatory Compliance

Standard Operating Procedures for the Conduct of Clinical Research

Developed to help clinical research sites meet the challenge of maintaining rigorous standards in a world of diminishing resources. The template has been expanded to include more procedures to assess study feasibility, recruit subjects and ensure regulatory compliance and is based on the Code of Federal Regulations and GCP Consolidated Guidelines.

Policies and Standard Operating Procedures for the Institutional Review Board

An efficient way for IRBs to document policies and procedures that reflect their organization's philosophies, standards and innovations while continuing to comply with federal regulations. The SOP template is based on the Code of Federal Regulations, guidance and ICH/GCP Consolidated Guideline and the Association for the Accreditation of Human Research Protection Program's (AAHRPP) standards for human subject protection.

Standard Operating Procedures for Good Clinical Practice by Sponsors of Clinical Trials

Developed to assist pharmaceutical and biotechnology companies maintain the quality performance and ethical conduct of clinical trials while adhering to U.S. federal regulations. The template contains 30 procedures addressing all Good Clinical Practice requirements and is based on FDA regulations and ICH guidelines.

Standard Operating Procedures for Good Clinical Practice by Sponsors of Medical Device Clinical Trials

Provides detailed SOPs to address specific requirements for medical device research practices to adhere to a discrete set of FDA regulations and guidance. Organizations that sponsor clinical research on new medical devices must implement procedures that comply with both Good Clinical Practice guidelines and federal regulations.

Medical Writing Services

Medical Writing Services

CenterWatch provides comprehensive medical writing and custom publishing services for pharmaceutical, biotech and contract research organizations to support their clinical development initiatives through post-approval marketing.

Medical Writing Services also has expanded offerings and expertise in the healthcare, academia and medical communications sectors.

Information Solutions and Content Licensing

Drugs in Clinical Trials Database

With more than 4,000 new investigational treatments in clinical trials worldwide, this database is updated weekly and is an effective resource for sponsors, CROs, research centers, service providers and analysts seeking to monitor drug performance, track competitors' development activity, identify development partners and clinical grant opportunities and analyze drug information for potential investments. Detailed drug profiles are completely searchable and include indications for use, current trial results, study phase status and manufacturer contact information.

Content Licensing

CenterWatch offers licensing of our database-driven and static-text content to provide companies with the latest in scientific clinical trial activity and drug development information using market intelligence and knowledge resources. Content can be offered as data feeds and co-branded to seamlessly integrate with a company's web site or Intranet. Our offerings include:

- Clinical Trials Listing Service™
- Drugs in Clinical Trials Database
- Recently Approved Drugs by the FDA
- New Medical Therapies™
- Patient Education
- Publication Content Portal

Business Development and Partnership Opportunities

Industry Provider Profile Pages

Industry Provider Profile Pages, located on centerwatch.com, create visibility for contract service providers to showcase their products and services online to the clinical trials community making it a useful and cost-effective way for providers to generate new business leads, increase exposure and reach a captive and targeted audience. Profile Pages are completely customizable and can include images and links to video presentations, demos and company documents.

Partnership Opportunities

CenterWatch has developed numerous partnerships and professional relationships with sponsors, CROs, health associations, niche providers and other organizations in order to better provide the clinical research community and patients with access to the most current and relevant industry, educational and patient-related information possible.

As market research experts, we also collaborate with organizations on various custom projects to conduct both broad and targeted industry-related surveys and to provide detailed data analysis about the clinical research industry.